SPAGYRICS

*The Alchemical Preparation of
Medicinal Essences, Tinctures,
and Elixirs*

Manfred M. Junius

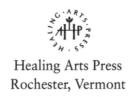

Healing Arts Press
Rochester, Vermont

Healing Arts Press
One Park Street
Rochester, Vermont 05767
www.HealingArtsPress.com

Healing Arts Press is a division of Inner Traditions International

Originally published in Italian under the title *Alchimia verde—Spagyrica vegetale* by Edizioni Mediter-
ranee, Rome.
The original Italian text was revised and enlarged by the author for a German edition published in 1982
under the title *Praktisches Hanbuch der Pflanzen-Alchemie* by Ansata-Verlag, Interlaken. The present
English translation is based on this German edition.

First U.S. edition published in 1985 by Inner Traditions under the title *The Practical Handbook of Plant
Alchemy.*
Second edition published in 1993 by Healing Arts Press.
Third edition published in 2007 by Healing Arts Press under the title *Spagyrics: The Alchemical Prepara-
tion of Medicinal Essences, Tinctures, and Elixirs.*

The English translation of the Aphorisms of the Circulatum Minus of Urbigerous has been reprinted
from the Golden Manuscript series with the kind permission of Frater Albertus and Paracelsus College
in Salt Lake City.

Note to the reader: *The book is intended as an informational guide. The remedies, approaches, and
techniques described herein are meant to supplement, and not to be a substitute for, professional medical
care or treatment. They should not be used to treat a serious ailment without prior consultation with a
qualified healthcare professional.*

Library of Congress Cataloging-in-Publication Data
Junius, Manfred M.
     [Alchimia verde--Spagyrica vegetale. English]
     Spagyrics : the alchemical preparation of medicinal essences, tinctures and elixirs / Manfred M.
Junius.—[3rd ed.]
     p. cm.
     Originally published: The practical handbook of plant alchemy. 1993.
     Includes bibliographical references and index.
     ISBN-13: 978-1-59477-179-8 (pbk.)
     ISBN-10: 1-59477-179-0 (pbk.)
     1. Materia medica, Vegetable. 2. Alchemy. I. Title.
RS164.J7613 2007
615'.321—dc22

                                         2007013911

ISBN of current title *Spagyrics:* ISBN-13: 978-1-59477-179-8; ISBN-10: 1-59477-179-0

Printed and bound in the United States

10 9 8 7 6

Design and Layout by Jonathan Desautels
This book was typeset in Sabon with Hathor Compress as a display typeface

CONTENTS

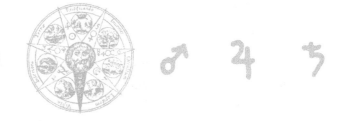

FOREWORD

The vast field of spagyrics presents itself rather like a mosaic that is only slowly completed by the collaboration of the reader.

—MANFRED JUNIUS

I am honored to write this foreword to this new edition and so present one of the key alchemical works of the twentieth century—*Spagyrics* by Manfred Junius. This book was first translated from the German *Praktisches handbuch der Pflanzen-Alchemie* and published in English in 1985 under the title *The Practical Handbook of Plant Alchemy*.

What most impressed me when I first read the book twenty-two years ago, and what continues to impress, was the generosity and directness of the material. As you read and re-read and begin to work your way through the processes given, you will begin to see the hand of a very skillful teacher.

The book outlines a coherent and true path. Starting with basic theories and simple effective processes, Manfred Junius builds to more complex spagyrical processes such as the *Circulatum Minus*. The Circulatum Minus is a solvent that can separate out, rather quickly, the principles of any fresh herb. He shows clearly how to obtain this unusual liquid using the techniques given in a seventeenth-century text. There is no one better qualified to do so as Manfred Junius was, perhaps, the first to recover this process and successfully make a Circulatum Minus—which indeed does some rather remarkable things. The book then gives a complete and very interesting primary text on working with wine. By the time you have worked through your collaboration with the processes given, you are more than ready to venture alone into this vast field of alchemy. And from this work, with grace, you will have realized in your heart that the real secret of alchemy is that there is no secret, no tricks, no special ingredient, only the work.

While *Spagyrics* is, by all appearances, a modest handbook—a "cookbook" some have even said, using a term that may seem to diminish the work—until you actually have to do the cooking, until you actually engage in the work, only then do you come to appreciate the scope and depth of this remarkable text. You won't find much discussion of the spiritual or inner work involved with alchemy in this book, no real in-depth discussion of "higher alchemical" practices, and this is perhaps as it should be, as these practices are based on initiation and cannot be taught through books. From discussions I've had with Manfred, I believe he would concur with the notion that if an individual would work within his or her own spiritual tradition, initiation would come. Although he was never very specific about the spiritual aspects of alchemy, he did urge one to a consideration of purpose as well as ethics. He would often say that the work is "karmically secure" if it is dedicated toward healing in particular and in helping others in general. When he wrote this book, he wrote it with the mind and heart of a healer. This comes across very clearly, as the book itself asks to be read with such a mind and such a heart.

Now, in 2007, we have a new edition for which I was delighted to assist in freshening the reproduction of the engravings from the alchemical literature. The illustrations and diagrams have been left as originally rendered by Manfred Junius and his hand-drawn symbols remain in the chapter about alchemical signs and symbols. Along with a new index to the content, I think this new edition is a balance of beauty, meaning, and history, serving well the purpose of the work at hand—to provide a handbook to the alchemical work with plants.

This work is not to be followed slavishly but listened to, experimented with. As gold tried in the fire remains pure gold, so it is with this work of Manfred Junius. Having been engaged in alchemical research and experimentation, I can attest that it all works and that all you need can be found here within these pages. The only thing missing is the agent to do the work: the heart, mind, and hands to bring it all to completion. The door to alchemy is literally in your hands.

BRIAN COTNOIR
WINTER SOLSTICE 2006

Brian Cotnoir is the author of *The Weiser Concise Guide to Alchemy*. He has studied alchemy for thirty-five years and was a contributor to *Parachemy,* the journal of Frater Albertus' Paracelsus Research Society. He first met Manfred Junius in 2000 at an alchemy conference in the Czech Republic.

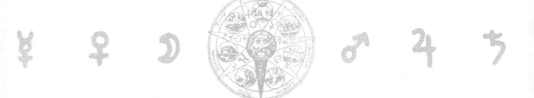

PREFACE

The renewed valuation of natural healing methods in our time has led to a steadily growing interest in medicinal plants and their classical—and thus also the spagyric—methods of preparation. The practice of spagyrics consists in the application of alchemical, or parachemical, findings and methods to the preparation of tinctures, essences, and other products from the medicinal plants at our disposal. This book aims to give the reader an understanding of these methods.

I have tried to present spagyrics holistically. Without knowledge of the conceptual world and background of spagyric thought, a mere practical methodology would be incomplete. The most important methods of preparation are discussed separately, while corresponding important textual passages are quoted in the original.

At the same time, as an experimental manual, this work will, it is hoped, stimulate the practice of spagyrics. By the very nature of our field, such a book can never be complete. Moreover, a certain inconsistency is hard to avoid. The vast field of spagyrics presents itself rather like a mosaic that is only slowly completed by the collaboration of the reader.

The lively response to the original Italian version induced me to enlarge this work in the German language, on which the present English translation is based. The bibliography contains the titles of further works that may later be consulted for advanced studies.

It is assumed that the reader has a fundamental knowledge of botanic medicine, or that he or she is willing to acquire it. For that reason, this book does not deal with individual medicinal plants. Several excellent works on this subject are easily available. (See the bibliography.)

In principle, spagyric preparations contain the curative powers of the plants used in each case, either integrally or partially. By further specific processes unique to spagyrics, these curative powers can be further potentized either all together or separately.

The hermetic terminology often strikes the uninitiated as strange and can easily lead to misunderstanding; one must therefore familiarize oneself with the often dramatic and always figurative language of this field, although it thereby loses much of its beauty and evocativeness. Anyone who walked into a laboratory supply store asking for suitable equipment for the "extraction of the Philosophical Principles" of plants, or for an "alembic for spirits," would be greeted by a perplexed look, unless the salesclerk happened to have a knowledge of spagyrics. An initiated spagyrist, however, would immediately understand the request and be able to make appropriate suggestions, for behind these terms that at first seem absurd are hidden clear concepts.

The classification of plants after the seven planets of antiquity may arouse reformatory urges in modern astrologers. Modern astrological research also takes into consideration the transsaturnians, and possibly still other influences and rhythms. Out of respect for the classical tradition, I have limited myself to the septenary. Besides, a distinction has to be made between the seven planetary *principles* as such and their planets.

In our time, parachemistry has become ever more accessible to the public and is today practiced in many countries. Medicines from the leading spagyric pharmaceutical companies as well as from good individual spagyrists are helping people throughout the world.

The bibliography of the Swiss edition retains several titles from the original Italian edition. Similarly, the acknowledgments expressed there are repeated here. Special thanks are due to Mr. Augusto Pancaldi, Ascona, friend and teacher of the author; to Professor Dr. Krishna Kumar, formerly of the Calabrian State University, today general manager of the Australerba Laboratories in Adelaide; and to the Āyurvedic physician Dr. Bhagwan Dash of New Delhi, also a much-revered teacher of the author. Thanks also to Hans Nintzel for his kind assistance in reading the English manuscript.

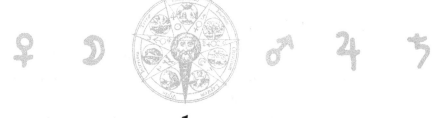

1
SPAGYRIA AND SPAGYRICS

Therefore, learn Alchimiam, otherwise called Spagyria,
which teaches you to separate the false from the true.

—PARACELSUS

In the word *spagyria* two Greek words are hidden: *spaō,* to draw out, to divide; and *ageirō,* to gather, to bind, to join. These two concepts form the foundation of every genuine alchemical work, hence the often-quoted phrase *"Solve et coagula, et habebis magisterium!"* (Dissolve and bind, and you will have the magistery).[1]

The alchemical work always takes place in three stages: (1) separation, (2) purification, and (3) cohobation (recombination, or the "chymical wedding"). In the spagyrist's view, these actions lead to an increase and a release of certain curative powers in the initial species.

Spagyric is the application of alchemical working methods to the production of medicaments.

When we learn that the famous physician Theophrastus Bombastus von Hohenheim, better known as Paracelsus (c. 1493–1541), prepared a large part of his famous medicines according to spagyric methods, we must thereby understand a very high level of the hermetic art. The latter has little in common with vulgar alchemy, which is often disparagingly called "the art of goldmaking."

The beginnings of this true hermetic art are to this day shrouded in obscurity. We know that the hermetic-spagyric method of preparation was known to many ancient cultures. In ancient China,[2] for instance, in India,[3] and among the ancient Egyptians,[4] we find important contributions to alchemical medicine. Between the ancient Indian and Chinese alchemy there exist many parallels. In India, alchemical preparations are part of the southern Indian *siddha* medicine, of Āyurvedic medicine and also of Unānī medicine, which came later to India through the Muslims and represents a further development of ancient Greek medicine.

The alchemy of the Western schools is chiefly based on the Egyptian tradition. In ancient Egypt, hermetism was taught in the temples of Memphis and Thebes. From the writings of Zosimos of Panopolis (Akhmin, A.D. 300) we learn that alchemy was practiced in Egypt under the supervision of kings and priests, and that divulging the secrets of this art was against the law.[5] The hermetic art was taught exclusively by oral transmission.

The Arabs were the chief agents for transmitting theoretical and practical alchemy to the Europeans, who then merged it with the Christian tradition.

Among the historically accessible European sources, special mention must be made of the writings of Paracelsus. Before the much older Indian and Chinese traditions became known in the West, the Paracelsian writings constituted the earliest information that could be dated with certainty. The dating of earlier texts, including many Oriental ones, is uncertain, and their authorship is elusive. The substructure of the whole alchemical world of ideas is strongly metaphorical and mythological, largely lacking the modern historical thinking that Westerners value so highly. It is no wonder, then, that many Western alchemists constantly refer to Paracelsus, and that several institutes bear his name.

In his book *Paragranum,* Paracelsus says: "The third foundation upon which medicine rests is alchemy. If the physician does not have good ability and experience in it, his art is in vain."

How do spagyric plant remedies differ from nonspagyric ones? Ordinary tinctures, infusions, decoctions, and the like, utilize in part the curative powers of the plants from which they are prepared. The spagyric preparation "opens" the plant and by its own process liberates stronger curative powers. It is in principle synergistic, and less interested in isolated pharmacologically active principles. We cannot do justice to the methodology of spagyrics if we measure it according to the standards of analytical chemistry or pharmacology, even if these sciences can explain in their own way part of the effects of spagyric remedies. Just as homeopathy has its own findings, experiences, and laws, which cannot be comprehended solely by the prevailing chemical-analytical knowledge, so, too, does spagyric insist on its own standards, for which it has its own conceptions and symbols. In the case of many of these conceptions and ideas we are dealing with analogies, which, however, prove to be extremely valuable, just as in traditional acupuncture.[6]

We must not consider spagyrics and alchemy as a whole merely a preliminary stage of the later scientific chemistry. It is rather another way of looking at nature and its powers. And as modern Western chemistry and medicine, at the latest since Virchow, broke completely with the chemical and medicinal arts of the past, many perceptions of spagyrics have remained closed to them. There exists a somewhat similar relation between chemistry and alchemy as between neurophysiology and acupuncture. Felix Mann, M.D., president of the Medical Acupuncture Society, who has striven for many years for a scientific explanation of acupuncture in the Western sense, writes in one of his books:

> What I have written . . . [in this work] might give the reader the impression, that there is little left to acupuncture, for I have demolished practically the whole of the traditional theoretical framework. This is far from being the case, for I practise acupuncture exclusively about 90% of my time, and I would not do so if I did not achieve *better* results than in practising Western medicine in the appropriate type of disease or dysfunction. There are, of course, many diseases where Western medicine is better than acupuncture.
>
> The crux of the matter is that I try to combine acupuncture with the principles of Western physiology, anatomy and medicine in

general. In some instances Chinese theory explains phenomena better than Western theory, and hence I treat the patient accordingly. I try to keep my feet in both camps, for there is much that is unknown to Western physiology that can in a certain way be explained by Chinese tradition, or at least enough of it can be explained to know how to treat a patient from an acupuncture point of view.[7]

We easily succumb to the temptation to judge the whole alchemical knowledge of the past by the criteria of the current stand of Western science, which leads to a distortion or an incomplete perception of genuine connections.

Analysis can never lead to a complete perception, because the whole is always greater than its parts. Thus, for instance, analytical examinations of old Italian master violins have never been able to unveil the secret of the famous violinmakers of Cremona. The whole scientific examination of the old violinmaking, including the analysis of the famous varnishes, could never lead to new heights of violinmaking, because it solely undertook the "solve" but not the "coagula." The quality of the master instruments of Stradivari and Guarneri del Gesù has remained unattainable to this day. I once asked a famous contemporary violinmaker, who could literally awaken an old instrument to new life, to tell me the "secret" of the old masters of Cremona. His reply was clear: "There are no secrets in the sense of tricks, as you might think. The 'secrets' consist of the true knowledge of natural laws and their bases, which the old masters understood better than we today."

It is similar with spagyrics. The spagyrist has to "stand in the light of nature," to quote once more from Paracelsus.

In this connection, a quotation from the *Ṛgveda* is here also cited: "The structure of pure knowledge—expression of the Veda—is contained in the immortal field of transcendental consciousness, in which all impulses of creative intelligence [or the laws of nature], which are responsible for the organization of the whole of creation, have their seat."[8]

Finally, a saying from an Indian guru of our age: "Knowledge is structured in consciousness."[9]

We rightly admire the amazing height of metallurgical knowledge in ancient India and China. The *bhasmas* of Indian Āyurvedic
medicine, which chemically are metallic oxides, have proved to be
excellent remedies in both ancient and modern times.[10] Thus, for example, *lohā-bhasma,* a specially prepared metallic oxide, does not show any
of the known side effects of many Western iron preparations and therefore causes neither constipation nor digestive troubles. It quickly enters
the bloodstream and raises the hemoglobin content, whereas many Western iron preparations can lead to gastric troubles and other side effects,
even when they are injected intravenously. These Āyurvedic *bhasmas* are
made by calcining metals (to which I shall refer later in detail), followed
by immersing them in plant juices. This process is repeated many times,
until the preparation has reached the desired condition.

Alchemists occasionally speak about an elevation *(exaltatio)* of the
basic substances. Spagyrists are of the opinion that these elevations liber-
ate specific energies. Let us consider two reproductions from "Sapientia
veterum philosophorum sive doctrina eorundem de summa et universali
medicina," a manuscript of the eighteenth century, preserved in Paris.[11]

In figure 1 we recognize a hermetically sealed flask, in which four
states of aggregation and a pelican are indicated. The exaltation takes
place in a pelican (see page 157), that is, in a reflux system.

Figure 2 shows the exalted essence: the volatile (white) is simultaneously above and below, right and left, likewise the fixed (dark). In the
center of the circle a phoenix is rising out of the fire, while the aura of
flames surrounding the flash denotes the now liberated energy in the
form of radiation. The states of aggregation are here united; the "circle
of clouds" is running its course.

To arrive at this release of higher energies, the alchemical art is
required. Let us listen to what Paracelsus has to say in this regard:

As Nature is extremely subtle and penetrating in her manifestations,
she cannot be used without the Art. Indeed, she does not produce
anything that is perfect in itself, but man must make it perfect, and
this perfecting is called alchemy. . . .

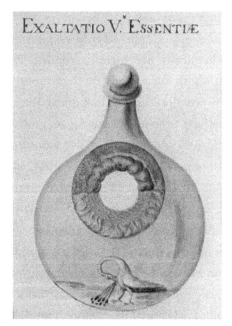

Fig. 1

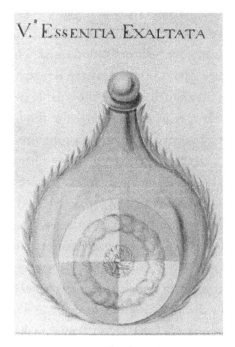

Fig. 2

And as medicine must not act without the participation of heaven, it must act together with it. Therefore you must treat it in order to free it from the Earth;[12] and as the latter is not ruled by heaven, it must be removed in the preparation of the medicine. When you have separated the medicine from the Earth, it obeys the will of the stars, that is, it will be guided by them. [*Paragranum*]

Whereas in the preparation of simple tinctures the plant residues are thrown out after the extraction, spagyric herbal preparations always contain the salts obtained through incineration and calcination of the plant residue. These are partly water-soluble and are leached from the calcined material with distilled water. By evaporating the water, one can make them visible. The nonwater-soluble salts are mostly (but not always!) rejected as Caput Mortuum (Death's Head) or *terra damnata* (damned earth), while the water-soluble ones go into the preparation as *Sal salis* (Salt of the salts). Experience has shown that these salts have great curative effects, and they are therefore also often used by themselves.

Like all alchemical methods of preparation, spagyrics considers the so-called three Philosophical Principles, also known as Essentials, the essential carriers of the curative powers. These three Essentials are designated as Mercury, Sulfur, and Salt. They must not be mistaken for the usual meaning of these words in present-day chemistry. By means of special processes, which we shall learn later, they are separated, cleansed (purification), and finally recombined (cohobation or chymical wedding).

For a long time modern Western pharmacology has been devoted to the investigation of single active substances that were, or are, extracted from the species. It has carried out the "solve," but only in rare cases the "coagula." Nevertheless, this modern research is absolutely valuable. It has made possible, for instance, the exact determination of critical amounts of certain substances and their specific weight, as well as many other qualitative-quantitative experiments. Through the pioneer work of nutritionists and naturopaths who had not made a complete break with the past but linked up with tradition, the holistic manufacture and dispensing of plant medicaments has gained ground once more. Even if some scientists have been holding on to extreme specialization up to today and have thereby largely lost the great synoptic view, science as a whole is nevertheless on the way to a new integral perspective. In this connection, many quotations can be cited. Here are a few of them:

> Our daily experience, down to the smallest detail, seems to be so much dovetailed into the large-scale features of the universe that it is practically impossible to consider the two as separate.[13]
>
> Modern physics teaches us that the "raw material" of the universe is an energy flow in fields of which matter represents only a manifestation. Einstein already said: "The field is the sole reality."[14]
>
> It was not possible to formulate the laws of the quantum theory without referring to consciousness.[15]

The exact definition of biochemical processes presents itself not only as a chemical but often also as an alchemical, or nuclear-chemical, problem. To understand, respectively to try to understand, the subtle effect of specific substances, we must become conversant with the concept of transmutation.

Let us begin with a personal experience of the author.

When, as a young student at an Indian university, I was obliged to eat in the Mensa, some food at first gave me trouble, especially the custom of eating citrus fruit, in particular grapefruit, with fairly large amounts of salt. Even fruit-juice beverages were often served salted. Aside from the omnipresent tea, the typical summer beverage was the dearly beloved *nimbū pānī,* a mixture of lemon juice, well water, and salt. Slowly I got used to many alien conceptions of nutrition, among others also the custom of always being served two small seeds in half a papaya fruit, instead of eating the fruit without seeds. When I inquired about the reason for this custom, approximately the following conversation developed:

"Why do we always find two seeds in the papaya? Is there any symbolic meaning?"

"The two seeds are good for your health. They contain substances that act favorably upon the digestive system during the digestion of the food. Always eat the seeds together with the fruit. We have our own traditional medicine and a precise science of nutrition. It is founded on insights that differ in many ways from your Western medicine. The word *Āyurveda* means 'science of life.' Āyurvedic medicine is one of the most successful systems of treatment by a precise science of nutrition, and a highly developed preventive medicine. One of its goals is to make the organism capable of resistance. Where your physicians proceed with antibiotics, often in cases where they are not necessary, the Āyurvedic physician would rather aim at an intensification of the defensive forces. He achieves this by restoring the balance of forces in the organism. It is like the combative sports: Whoever has balance, stands firm. Where stability loses equilibrium, lability ensues, as in judo. By this I do not mean to say anything against your medicine, which is excellent in surgery and technology. Indeed, every system has its place, and none is quite complete without the other. Or take Unānī medicine. The word *Unānī* means 'Greek,' properly speaking, 'Ionic.' This system is akin to your classical medicine, Hippocrates and others. The Muslims brought it to our country.

"There are many processes in our organism—and I beg you to understand this word in a much wider sense than you are perhaps used to—which the official Western medicine does not know. The *prāṇa* energy of the breath and the *nāḍīs*, for example, are unknown to Western medicine, likewise the meridians of Chinese medicine. Breathing is not only oxygen absorption. Still quite different energies and transformations of energy are involved. My father was a *vaidya* [Āyurvedic physician] in Allahabad. You will see that it will not be long before Āyurvedic medicine is also taught at our modern universities."[16]

"That may be so. But perhaps you could explain to me why fruit and lemonade are always salted here. I am always advised to drink a great deal here in India, as much liquid evaporates through the skin in the heat. Is salt meant to bind the water in the body? Or to replace the salts lost with the liquid?"

"It is not quite so simple. We cannot simply replace certain salts essential to life with table salt or with natural sea salt. Salt brings a certain freshness. It protects you from exhaustion in great heat. Wheat, for instance, is cool and sweet by nature, and its digestive product is sweet. This water buffalo's milk here is fat and cool. According to the Āyurveda, there are eight different kinds of honey, for example, fresh sweet honey, astringent honey, light and cool honey, and so on. This fruit here (papaya) is sweet, heavy, appetizing, and it reduces *pitta*. What *pitta* (gall) means, I'll explain to you when the time comes."

"But how can I feel fresh when this sharp salt is in my body?"

"It produces many effects in the organism. Do take up the Indian science of nutrition and medicine. I advise you in good faith to become accustomed to our eating and drinking habits."

It *was* good advice. During half of my life in India, I was never seriously ill, which may be attributed to a healthy way of life, adapted to Indian conditions and the Āyurveda.

For a long time I could not find a completely satisfactory explanation for the frequent use of salt. The often-heard assertion that it was merely a replacement for the secretion of lost salts and substances did not satisfy me, if only for the reason that sea salt does not contain all physiologically necessary salts and trace elements. Only the study of alchemy—more exactly, of biological transmutations—could throw some light upon the problem. Now a few words about this.

When the biologist Dr. L. C. Kervran was on official mission in the Sahara in 1959, he observed that those technicians and workmen who were preserved from heatstroke and exhaustion, even at enormous temperatures and while working intensely, all took large amounts of sea salt, mostly in the form of tablets. (These tablets had also been distributed to the British armed forces in India during the colonial times.) Repeated investigations by Dr. Kervran, which were also confirmed by other researchers, proved that the perspiration of the workers contained a very high percentage of potassium after taking the salt tablets. Table salt, however, is sodium chloride, not potassium. What had happened to the sodium?

It had changed into potassium within the organism and could later be detected in the perspiration in the already mentioned high amounts. This process uses up calories. ("Salt brings a certain freshness. It protects you from exhaustion in great heat.") Hence the cooling effect, an endothermic process.

Dr. Kervran formulated this process as follows:

$$_{11}^{23}\text{Na} + {_8^{16}}\text{O} = {_{19}^{39}}\text{K}$$

This formula represents the substantial side of the progress; the energy factor is not discernible in it.

Such nuclear-chemical formulas—we can call them "alchemical" or "parachemical" formulas—have not been in use for very long. The ancient masters used other symbols, among them often very impressive, highly dramatic images, such as dragons with or without wings, red and green lions, snakes, crows, eagles, toads, salamanders, flowers, trees, chains, and gods and goddesses. We are prone today to express many parachemical processes in nuclear-chemical formulas, which were of course unknown to the ancient masters. But we should not overlook the fact that the concrete and metaphorical language of the alchemists is not only of great beauty but also very evocative and precise. C. G. Jung, who was at first confused by the language of alchemistic treatises, later, after advanced studies, pointed out the extraordinary coherence and precision of alchemistic concepts and formulations—true, always from the viewpoint of the psychologist. Practical alchemy remained closed to him.

It was not so long ago that official chemistry denied the possibility of transformation of the elements; just for the same reason it spoke of basic substances. Modern research has forced chemistry to change its formulations, because the possibility of transmuting one element into another has been proved experimentally.

We shall now briefly refresh our nuclear-chemical knowledge.

Transmutation means the transformation of one element into another. A radioactive element is constantly transmuting. The atoms give off particles, whereby the number of protons changes and a new element is formed. This process continues until a stable element is formed, for instance, lead. Science distinguishes between three kinds of nuclear changes: fission, fusion, and transmutation.

In fission (splitting), the nucleus splits into two nuclei; in fusion (joining together), two or several nuclei combine into a heavier nucleus. (Here, too, the famous sentence applies: *Solve et coagula, et habebis magisterium.*) In the course of a transmutation (transformation), a radioactive element disintegrates through regular emission of particles. Every element can be made radioactive by bombarding it with alpha particles or neutrons. In this way, the element changes into a radioactive "isotope."

In alchemy, the concept of transmutation is simply identical with every transformation of elements.

In classical alchemistic texts, we also find the word *projection.* The transformation of a substance is done according to an alchemical method by throwing upon it—that is, "projecting"—a specific active principle. In this sense the bombardment of matter with accelerated particles that cause a transmutation can also be called a modern form of projection. Since the transmuted matter changes color, classical alchemy also speaks of "tingeing."

Ernest Rutherford was the first scientist to succeed in bringing about an artificial transmutation of elements in the laboratory in the modern scientific meaning. By means of a helium nucleus (an alpha particle), he transmuted a nitrogen nucleus into an oxygen isotope and hydrogen after the formula:

$$_{7}^{14}N + {_{2}^{4}He} \mapsto {_{8}^{17}O} + {_{1}^{1}H}$$

Scientific knowledge and formulation of transmutation led to a change in the concept of elements. "Element" in the modern meaning stands for a pure substance whose constituent atoms are all of the same kind. Elements are homogeneous systems of a constant, nonvariable combination that cannot be divided by chemical means.

We shall later see that the concept of elements in alchemy is totally different and rather resembles a state, since alchemy does not recognize stability in the matter found in the realms of nature. In nature, nothing but change is stable, and nature itself represents a constantly occurring alchemy.

A chemical element, therefore, is a body composed of atoms of one kind. Each of these atoms consists of a nucleus with the same number of protons, respectively also neutrons, and an "orbit" or "shell" of "revolving" electrons whose number is identical with that of the protons. This atomic model goes back to Ernest Rutherford and Niels Bohr and has been able to survive until today on the strength of its clarity, at least among chemists, while physicists are especially interested in the still more minute building stones of matter, which they provisionally call "elementary particles." In modern nuclear physics, the concepts of the elementary particles are undergoing changes that often border on the limits of our imagination.

Let us for the moment remain with our already somewhat old-fashioned proton-electron-neutron model.

Protons have a positive charge, electrons a negative, neutrons are neutral. If an atom has more neutrons in its nucleus than protons, its atomic weight is higher. Such an atom is called an isotope. Isotopes are atoms of an identical chemical but of a higher atomic weight owing to the presence of neutrons. In this way, for instance, exist the heavy hydrogens. The "normal" hydrogen, atomic weight 1.008, consists of one proton and one electron; deuterium, atomic weight 2.016, has one neutron in addition; the still heavier tritium, atomic weight 3.024, has two neutrons in addition.

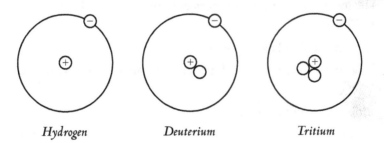

Hydrogen   *Deuterium*   *Tritium*

In our abovementioned formulas, the upper number, called the mass number, indicates the sum of the number of protons and neutrons (if those are present), while the lower represents the number of electrons. We can now easily understand Kervran's formula of the transformation of sodium into potassium: The nucleus of the sodium isotope with 11 protons and 12 neutrons fuses with the oxygen nucleus, which consists of 8 protons and 8 neutrons. The electrons are likewise added. The result is a new atom with a nucleus consisting of 19 protons (11 + 8) and 20 neutrons (12 + 8), around which 19 electrons (11 + 8) revolve, which is a potassium isotope.

That this kind of transmutation, about which many scientists are still skeptical, represents a certain heat regulation of the organism, seems also to be confirmed by other observations.

In tropical climates, the potassium content in human urine rises considerably in proportion to the sodium content, especially in the course of physical work.

We will here mention yet another example of biological transmutation. According to the classical Doctrine of Signatures (see chapter 6), horsetail (the most frequently used species, *Equisetum arvense*) is considered to be ruled by Saturn. Among other organs, this plant in particular rules the bone structure and the mineral processes in the organism. Horsetail has a corrective effect in cases of demineralization of the bones, as also in general. (See the works of Leclerc, Renon, Kobert, Kahle, Willfort, and others.) Horsetail corrects and maintains the organic calcium equilibrium. This ability rests especially upon the transmutation of silicon into calcium.

The most important substances contained in field horsetail are:

1. Silicic acid in large amounts
2. Equisetic acid (an acid proper to the species, with a diuretic effect)
3. Equisetonin (a saponin)
4. Mucic acid

5. Malic acid
6. Oxalic acid
7. Iron
8. Magnesium
9. Manganese
10. Potassium
11. Sodium
12. Aluminum
13. Calcium
14. Phosphorus
15. Glucosides
16. Antivitamin (in the spores; the antivitamin has the ability to decompose vitamin B1, thiamine)
17. Dimethylsulfon
18. Vitamin C (in the fresh plant)
19. Phytostearin
20. Resin
21. A substance that prevents coagulating and floats on the juice of the plant
22. A coagulating substance in the sediment of the juice
23. An alkali not yet clearly defined
24. Equisetin, an alkaloid caused by a fungus *(Ustilago Equiseti)* that gives the plant its typical brown spots. If a content of equisetin is to be avoided, the plant must be harvested before it is attacked by the fungus.

Young plants contain less silicic acid than full-grown species. The younger plants, however, contain more soluble silicic acid than the older ones, whereby we have to bear in mind that soluble silicic acid has a greater therapeutic value.

According to information from the Firma Staufen Pharma company, the quantitative analysis of a horsetail species is as follows:[17]

Silicic acid: 62.11%

Chlorine: 0.70%

Sulfuric acid: 4.67%

Phosphoric acid: 2.12%

Sulfur: 4.03%

Carbonic acid: 0.59%

Potassium: 2.88%

Sodium: 0.67%

Magnesium: 1.53%

Calcium: 15.40%

Iron: 2.19%

Impressive is the high content in silicic acid, which is practically four times the calcium content. How then can the strongly balancing effect of the calcium content in the organism be explained? According to Kervran, the calcium content of the organism is especially maintained by the processes of transmutation. Here now follow the corresponding formulas:

$$1. \quad {}^{39}_{19}K + {}^{1}_{1}H = {}^{40}_{20}Ca$$

$$2. \quad {}^{24}_{12}Mg + {}^{16}_{8}O = {}^{40}_{20}Ca$$

$$3. \quad {}^{28}_{14}Si + {}^{12}_{6}C = {}^{40}_{20}Ca$$

The last of these formulas explains the process. In this connection, a remark by the American nutritionist Dr. Paavo Airola regarding osteoporosis is interesting.[18] An abnormal porosity of the bones of older people is usually due to deficient nutrition, especially a lack of vitamins and minerals. A prolonged treatment with cortisone can also end in osteoporosis, as it leads to a reduction of the intake of calcium through the intestines and also blocks the formation of bone substance. Dr. Airola remarks that, in Dr. Kervran's view, it is not advisable to give food rich in vitamins or supplementary calcium in cases of osteoporosis, calcium deficiency, or decalcification. Kervran instead suggests the intake of organic silicic acid, magnesium, and potassium as a more effective way to improve the mineral economy and to add calcium to the bones and tissues. By the process of biological transmutation, the silicon of the silicic acid in the body is changed into easily assimilable calcium. Kervran especially recommends horsetail tea.

In his book on biological transmutation, Kervran remarks that organic silicic acid is recommendable for human beings, while mineral silicic acid has the opposite effect: it decalcifies.[19]

These pointers must suffice for the moment. To the interested reader, the writings of Kervran and Vitofranceschi, mentioned in the bibliography of this work, are recommended.

In connection with the renewed evaluation of the possibilities of transmutation, I will also mention the much-discussed experiment of the Gesellschaft für Schwerionenforschung (Society for Research in Heavy Ions) in Darmstadt.

In 1977, a plate of uranium was bombarded with uranium ions that had been accelerated to a speed of 1.8 billion electron volts. With these energies a total fusion of two uranium nuclei does not yet occur, but only a few protons and neutrons are exchanged between the nuclei. This exchange increases with the growing energy of the projectiles, and in the subsequent (radiochemical) analysis the presence of gold was confirmed. When one of two uranium nuclei changes into a gold nucleus, the reaction partner changes into a nucleus of element 105 (uranium has the atomic number 92, gold 79; the difference is 13; 92 + 13 = 105). Such elements are unstable, however, and quickly disintegrated through nuclear fission.

The classical masters of alchemy did not make use of these enormously high momentary energies but used extremely subtle energies, such as those of the human organism. On the other hand, many alchemical processes proceed with infinite slowness. Works over many years and even decades are not unusual. Many scientists insist that transmutations are only possible with enormous expenditure of energy, but that they then occur with high speed. Why should it not be possible to achieve transmutations with lower energies but with a greater loss of time? Is it perhaps as with a pulley: either "much expenditure of energy and little time, or little expenditure of energy and much time"? Besides, how can the corresponding energies be measured, especially when they are not even known?

The old masters recommend that we always follow Nature and let her do the work of her own, like a farmer. The closeness of alchemy to agriculture has often been emphasized, and there were alchemists who assumed the nickname "Agricola." Figure 3 shows an engraving from Michael Maier's famous work *Atalanta Fugiens,* which indicates that the alchemist must follow the steps of Nature and light up her ways.

It is important for us to remember that the possibility of transmutation is a scientifically proven fact and in no way a creation of fancy. The dispute centers on the means, not on the fact as such. It was transmutation that made possible the appearance of the whole of matter at all. In the view of science, from the hydrogen that came out of the "Big Bang," ever heavier elements developed with the birth and death of generations of stars in about seven billion years. If we speak of matter as frozen light out of the Big Bang, we can also say: *In principio erat hydrogenium*—in the beginning was hydrogen, which is the most heat-related substance in the view of parachemistry.

Let us now return to spagyrics. For the preparation of spagyric remedies, only healthy medicinal plants are used, which have grown without artificial fertilizer. Likewise, it is best to use pure spring water. In addition, the spagyrist often considers the position of the planets and the planets as so-called horary (or hourly) rulers.

We shall once again quote Paracelsus in this connection:

Thus your medicine must bear its fruits as the summer bears its fruits. You must know that the summer does this with the help of the stars, not without them. If the stars are able to do this, you must

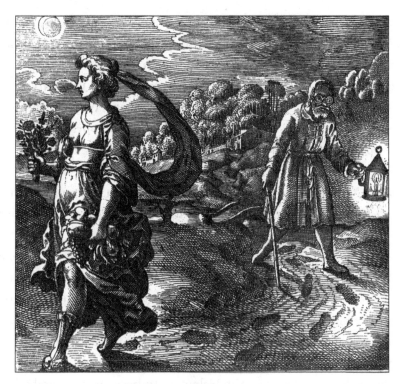

Fig. 3

"To him/who is dealing with chymics,/let Nature be reason/experience and reading/like a guide/staff/glasses and lamp."

know how the medicine is prepared in this way and that it is ruled by the stars. For it is they that complete the work of the physician. And since it is they that act, the medicine must be understood, classified, and adjusted according to their influence. . . . Therefore, one has to understand that the medicine must be prepared in the stars and that the stars become the medicine.   [*Paragranum*]

With the gradual advance of materialism and the spreading notion of the static concept of the element in official chemistry, alchemy lost increasingly more ground, although it was still prospering in the seventeenth century.

In the nineteenth century, the German physician Carl Friedrich Zimpel, M.D., Ph.D. (1800–1878), began a new production of spagyric medicaments. This widely traveled and learned man had originally been an engineer. He devoted himself late in life to the study of medicine and acquired a doctorate in philosophy and medicine. He was awarded the Prussian gold medal for art and science and was an honorary member of the Mineralogical Society of the University of Jena. In 1849, he established himself in London as a homeopathic physician. Zimpel devoted himself intensively to the study of the works of Paracelsus and Glauber. Gradually, he developed an important production, known today as Müller-Göppingen, with the special division of Staufen Pharma, a high-level, internationally known manufacturing firm, whose products are today available in many countries of the world.

Meanwhile, the research of Jung also led to a new valuation of alchemistic texts and concepts from the viewpoint of the psychologist. Jung recognized in the alchemical tradition a philosophical system of great coherence and persuasive power. In the meantime, many classical texts have been reprinted, in connection with which the attitude of the publishers vacillates strongly. Available, for instance, are the works of Paracelsus, Basilius Valentinus, Glauber, Van Helmont, Andreas Libavius, and others.

In 1921, Alexander von Bernus founded the Soluna Laboratory, formerly Stift Neuberg in Heidelberg. After a brief stay in Stuttgart, the institute moved to Castle Donaumünster in Donauwörth. Alexander von Bernus's book *Alchymie und Heilkunst* is warmly recommended to every reader. Now as ever, the Soluna Laboratory produces a large number of spagyric remedies.

The Phoenix Laboratory in Bondorf, which produces a number of reliable medicaments after the Paracelsus method, and the firm Naturwaren GmbH Dr. rer. nat. Peter Theiss in Homburg must also be mentioned in this connection.

In Salt Lake City, Utah, Frater Albertus (Dr. Albert Riedel) founded the present Paracelsus College, which has issued from the Paracelsus Research Society. Fra Albertus is one of the best-known representatives of alchemy in our time. His lectures in many countries have given a number of participants their first access to alchemy, even if some of them later preferred to work on their own.

In Switzerland, Augusto Pancaldi, friend and teacher of the author, is active. Pancaldi's students are working quietly in several countries.

In Australia, several alchemists are working assiduously. Here, where nature with its great wealth in gold and minerals has so clearly traced out the way, much will still develop, not least through the influence of the tradition of many cultures from East and West. Windmill in Victoria manufactures spagyric products, likewise Australerba in Adelaide, with its first-rate Integral Plant Elixirs, which are offered as practical herb teas. To this we must add a series of popular herb wines, a series of efficacious herb and honey compounds and tonics, as well as a number of hearty herb honeys that correspond to the Old Italian *melitti*. The honeys, which are also very much liked by children, are first-grade varieties from the vast, sun-drenched Australian countryside, enriched by spagyric herbal preparations. Australerba has done pioneering work with its products, which are today available on the entire Australian continent and overseas.

There exist many different methods of preparation of spagyric remedies. I shall deal with a large number of them in the present work. Some are relatively simple, others extremely complicated. Over and beyond this, the reader is meant to be stimulated into doing his or her own research and experimentation, and studying the classical texts.

Today, the issue at stake is the reexamination of the treasure of spagyrics regarding its mode of operation and to rid it of false claims. Not everything in the thousands of alchemistic treatises is genuine. In addition, often misconceptions form the basis of genuine processes; but misconceptions are also found in official school learning. To examine the tradition and the remedies, to take up further research with new starting points of thought, to respect the true and to separate the false in tradition—these are the commands of the hour. In this sense, too, the spagyric work should be an art that separates the false from the genuine. Let this idea of Paracelsus's be voiced once again at the end of the first chapter.

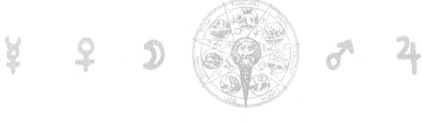

2
ADVICE OF
BASILIUS VALENTINUS

In this my consideration, I have actually found five
points, which are the noblest and which all seekers of
wisdom and lovers of the Art are in duty bound to inquire
into. First, there is the invocation of God; second, the
consideration of nature; third, the true unadulterated
preparation; fourth, the application; and fifth, the useful-
ness. These five points, then, every chymicus and true
alchymist must know how to consider and recognize. For
otherwise, without it, he cannot be perfect nor be com-
pletely recognized as a true spagirum.

—FROM THE *TRIUMPHAL*
CHARIOT OF ANTIMONY

The study and practice of alchemy are based on modesty, patience, seriousness, and determination. The higher alchemical practice can only be transmitted through the personal directions of a qualified teacher. Whoever reads the classical texts without a corresponding preparation and complement will understand little or nothing. Just like music, the alchemical art cannot be learned solely from books.

Fundamentally, alchemy will always remain an art built on personal initiation. We know little about the person of Basilius Valentinus. By his own testimony, he was a Benedictine monk.

Among his chymical writings we find the particularly important works *The Twelve Keys of Hermetic Philosophy* and the *Triumphal Chariot of Antimony.* Whether Basilius was an alchemist of the sixteenth century or whether he lived earlier is not of concern to us here. What is important is that we are dealing with an undisputed authority on alchemy.

Let us now turn to his five points of advice. The invocation of God is for every spagyrist the beginning and end, the alpha and omega of every intention and every action, and nothing is ever begun without it. In the classical texts some of these prayers have come down to us, which allow us to recognize the religious attitude of their author in each case. Here is an invocation by Nicolas Flamel, who was an eminent alchemist of the fourteenth and fifteenth centuries:

> Almighty, eternal God, Father of Light, from Whom all good things and perfect gifts come to us, I beg You, for the sake of Your infinite mercy, let me recognize Your eternal wisdom, that which surrounds Your throne, which has created and made everything, which guides and maintains everything. Send it to me from Heaven, Your sanctuary, and from the throne, Your glory, that it may enter me and work within me. [For] it is the mistress of all heavenly and secret arts, which opens up the knowledge of and insight into all things. Grant that it may accompany me in all my works, so that, strengthened by its spirit, I may receive the true insight and advance without error in the noble Art to which I have dedicated my life, in the exploration of the Philosopher's Stone, which You have hidden from the world but whose discovery You grant to Your elect. That I may happily begin, continue, and perfect this great work which I am called to accomplish on this earth, and that I may ever rejoice in it. For this I entreat You through Jesus Christ, the celestial Stone, pillar of the marvelous, founded for eternity, who determines and rules with You. Amen.

Nicolas Flamel asks for the right illumination, the right elevation and structuring of his consciousness, for the right wisdom that Forms the foundation of being.

And here a plain prayer of Paracelsus:

O Holy Spirit, show me what I do not know, and teach me what I cannot do, and give me what I do not have. Grant that You, O Holy Spirit, may dwell within my five senses; with the seven gifts You are to gift me, and I shall have Your divine peace. O Holy Spirit! Teach me and show me, so that I may live rightly with God and my neighbor.

What does Basilius Valentinus mean by "Consideration of Nature"? We shall let him speak for himself:

This true invocation of God is now followed by the consideration of every thing in the right order; this means that everything must be well considered in the beginning, namely the circumstances of every thing, what is its matter and form, from what it has taken its effect, by what it was infused and implanted, also how it was generated by the sideric, made by the elements, and was born and given form by the three principles. Likewise, how the body of anything can again be reversed, that is, dissolved into its Primam Materiam, or prime matter, as I have already discussed in various ways in my other writings, so that the ultima materia can again become the Prima Materia, and the Prima Materia again the ultima materia. . . .

This then is Theoria, namely, to fathom that which is visible and tangible and also has a temporal, formal nature, showing how to perfect it by its separation, so that every Corpus can tell us of its use, what is latent in it, good or bad, poison or medicine, how the unhealthy is to be separated from the healthy, also how to effect its Anatomia, and to carry out its destruction and breaking up, so that justo titulo, without wrong and sophistry, Purum ab Impuro can be separated, which separation can now be done by various manual operations, different ways and means, of which some are generally known but others not: such as Calcination, Sublimation, Reverberation, Circulation, Putrefaction, Digestion, Distillation, Cohobation, Fixation and the like, which grades are always discovered, learned, investigated, and revealed one after another in the course of the work, by which becomes known what is fixed and unfixed, what is white, black, red, blue, or green, and so forth, so that the artist may proceed in the right way and properly apply the consideration. . . .

Basilius calls upon us to meditate thoroughly on the matter and processes before acting.

What then is meant by "the true and unadulterated preparation"? After the theoretical reflection on things, the practical preparation follows, which requires the right attitude, devotion, and a corresponding skill. The manual work is added to the right knowledge, and in this way the work planned becomes a reality:

When then the consideration of everything has been rightly undertaken, which, as mentioned before, is nothing but Theoria, it is followed by the right, true preparation, which preparation must be done through manual work, so that something factual and real may follow afterward. Out of the preparation arises knowledge, namely such knowledge by which one can obtain the basis and opportunities for medicines.

The manual work is done through diligent application. Knowledge, however, is founded on experience. Anatomia is the right judge of both, enabling us to recognize the difference between the two. Manual work shows how all things can be made and prepared notoria, demonstrably and visibly; knowledge, however, brings to light practical methods and the right, true, and unadulterated basis from which a true Practicus can grow, and it is nothing but a confirmation that manual work reveals something good and has brought forth and demonstrated the hidden secret nature thereof for the good.

Now the right use:

When now your preparation has been made, namely the separation of the good from the bad, which must be done by the opening, you must thereafter take care of the proportion of weight, that you do not take too much or too little of a thing, which you may note and observe by the effect, whether the medicine is too strong or too gentle, likewise if it tends to be useful or harmful. A physician should know this beforehand and have an understanding of it, if he does not wish to "make a new graveyard," together with the loss and damnation of his soul and the decline of his good name.

And finally the usefulness:

After the remedy has begun to spread to all members of the body in order to seek out the infirmity for which it is prescribed and used, there finally follows its usefulness as the last thing whereby is recognized what good the remedy has contributed. For a thing or medicine may well be harmful and not helpful, which would affect the disease adversely and be a poison rather than a medicine for health.

Therefore, each must pay careful attention to the usefulness, noting and recording it, so that this usefulness is not forgotten but may also be applied to others.

Prior to every practical work, the theory must be understood. We are asked to repeatedly read carefully through the corresponding texts and to meditate on them.

Ora, lege, lege, lege, relege, labora, et invenies: pray, read, read, read, read once again, work, and you will find. This sentence is on the fourteenth plate of the *Mute Book (Mutus Liber)*, which is entirely done in the form of pictures and was first published in 1677 in La Rochelle.

Let us now consider two engravings. The first (figure 4) is from the collection of texts *Musaeum Hermeticum* (Frankfurt, 1678; reprint,

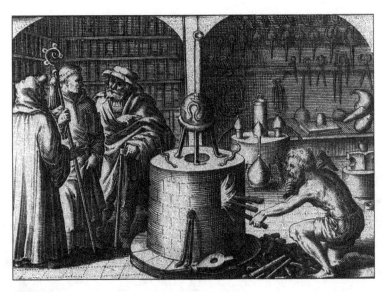

Fig. 4

Graz, 1970). The engraving shows that the theory (the library) and the practice (the laboratory) must go hand in hand to be successful in alchemy. We see three masters of the hermetic art: the Benedictine monk Basilius Valentinus, the abbot Cremerus of Westminster, and the Englishman Thomas Norton, author of the *Ordinall of Alchemy*. The last-named is pointing to the furnace on which an alchemical process is taking place. In the glass flask we recognize a winged snake, symbol of a volatile corrosive substance. The laboratory is symbolically represented as the forge of the god Vulcan. The god himself is serving the three masters by providing the furnace with wood for the fire.

The second engraving (figure 5) is from the collection *Amphitheatrum Sapientiae Aeternae* of the physician and alchemist Heinrich Khunrath (1560–1605). The draftsman of this particularly beautiful engraving is Hans Fredemann Vries; the engraver is Paulus van der Doost. The picture represents Khunrath's motto: "Persevering—Praying—Working." To the left we see an oratorium, a kind of prayer tent. The text on the plate in the tent reads: "Do not speak about God without the light." On the table there are books, symbolic drawings, and writing utensils. To the right is the laboratory. The two columns bear the inscriptions *Ratio* and

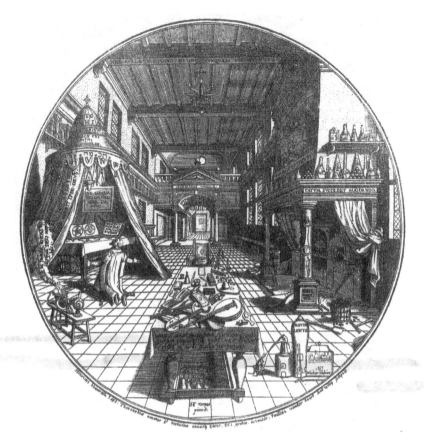

Fig. 5

Experientia, Reason and Experience. A distillation is just taking place, which separates "Soul" and "Spirit" (♀ and ☿). On the furnace we recognize the words *Festina lente* (Make haste slowly). In the center of the picture we see musical instruments,[20] symbols of the harmonic order of the world and the Art. The inscription reads: "The sacred music chases troubles and evil spirits away, because the Spirit of God sings with joy in the heart where the holy joy dwells." The door in the center of the picture points to the goal. It is far away, and outside it is light. The text on the archway reads: *Dormiens vigila* (While asleep, stay awake).

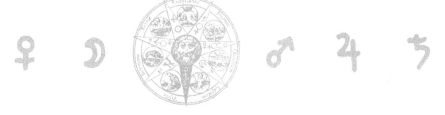

3
THE THREE PHILOSOPHICAL PRINCIPLES AND THE ELEMENTS

According to the alchemistic conception, the entire manifestation of matter is maintained through the cooperation of three Philosophical Principles, which are also called the Three Essentials or the Three Substances.

The different proportion of the three substances in the countless forms of manifestation of matter accounts for their multiplicity. For this reason, the various materially existing things are sometimes also called Mixta (mixtures). A metal, for instance, is a Mixtum, likewise a plant. In this way specific proportions of the Three Substances, or the Philosophical Principles or Essentials, form the basis of every chemical (not alchemical) element.

The three Philosophical Principles form a unity in the triad, although they are different from one another.

In alchemistic terminology these Principles are designated as Sulfur, Mercury, and Salt. These names are not to be mistaken for their usual meaning in the language of chemistry. Alchemical Sulfur is not the chemical element sulfur (S); likewise, the alchemical Mercury must not be regarded as identical with the metal quicksilver (Hg). It is not at all a question of metals, because metals are themselves composed of the three Philosophical Principles. If alchemists speak of sulfur and quicksilver in the metals, it does not mean that metals are considered mercury sulfates.

In the alchemical terminology the meaning is as follows:

Mercury: The principle of life, or the vital power, the spirit (in the sense of "spirit of life"), the waters of life, further, the volatile, the etheric. In the Indian tradition, Mercury is also called *prāṇa.* Mercury is considered anonymous and not conscious. It represents the feminine or passive principle.

Sulfur: The soul, consciousness, designated as *ātman* or *ātma* in the Indian tradition, that is, in the sense of *jīvātman,* the individual soul (also called the central point in consciousness), and also sometimes in the sense of universal Sulfur, that is, the World Soul *(paramātman).* Sulfur is always conscious and never anonymous. In the Indian Sāṁkhya philosophy the word *prāṇa* is always used in the sense of soul, but that is a peculiarity of *that* philosophical system. Furthermore, Sulfur is the fiery, radiant, burning, and masculine or active principle.

Salt (or sal): The solid, the body, the vehicle, matter in the sense proper.

From the aforesaid we can recognize that the designations *spirit* and *soul* are here used with another meaning than they have in the anthroposophical formulation, for instance, where spirit is consciousness and the soul is considered as living and mediating between spirit and body. We are here dealing with a difference in linguistic usage and not necessarily with a philosophical problem. The expression "life spirit" is an absolutely familiar concept for many readers trained in Western occult traditions.

The spirit (Mercury) in the alchemical sense is considered feminine. It is supple and plastic, but it can also have a corrosive effect. Arabian cosmologists use the term *rūḥ* (Hebrew *ruaḥ*), which also signifies the motion of the air or the living breath (Sanskrit *prāṇa*). The word is akin to the Arabic word *rīḥ* (air). Living creatures inhale the vital force with the air, so that it can nourish the subtler bodies or organs. Hence the Indian breathing technique known as *prāṇayāma*.

According to the Arabian philosopher and physician Averroës, the vital power is present in interstellar space as a substance. By specific breathing processes it can be assimilated, then transformed into life in the heart. This formulation brings back to mind the concept of ether in space. In the Indian tradition, it is called *ākāśa* (space or ether).

According to the Chinese conception, the vital power is differentiated into many further single vital forces, which are called different forms of *chi*. They are changing constantly, combine anew, are striving toward each other and again away from each other, and flow through organisms in various forms. *Chi* is elastic, moldable, adaptable. In breathing, in the Chinese view, cosmic energy mingles with the energies carried to the lungs from the spleen (and from other organs by way of the latter). This composite energy now flows in the meridian system in the point *(chung-fu)* known as Lung 1.

In the body, the Mercury principle is especially strong in the blood and the semen as also in the breath and the heart. In Indian alchemy, Mercury is also said to be the semen of Śiva. Śiva, God as the creator, transformer, and destroyer (so that something new can be created) is the Lord of alchemy and the cause of every transmutation.

Sulfur, or the soul, is the masculine principle. If Mercury is occasionally called the Moon, the lunar, or Diana, Sulfur is the Sun, the solar, Apollo, the original potency, the formative principle, the active, the principle of the "invisible fire," and also of love.

Let us now consider an engraving (figure 6) from the *Viridarium Chymicum* (Frankfurt, 1624). The triangle standing on its point represents the three Philosophical Principles. To the old man's left we see the inscription *Spiritus*. Here is the volatile (the bird opening its wings). We also recognize the Moon, the feminine principle. This corner represents Mercury. To the old man's right we recognize the inscription *Anima*. We also see the Sun, the masculine principle, and the salamander, symbol of the fiery factor. This corner represents Sulfur.

Sulfur and Mercury together form the law of polarity. In the lower

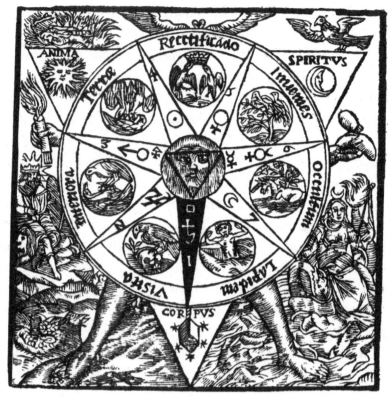

Fig. 6

vertex of the triangle we see a cube, the symbol of matter, surrounded by stars. The stars are the gigantic laboratories in which matter is developed. The cube signifies the corporeal and material pure and simple. As matter rests on the working together of polarized forces, it is neutral. The lower corner of the triangle represents Sal (Salt).

In the old man's right hand, on the Sulfur side, we see a torch, symbolizing fire, light, and warmth. In his left hand the old man is holding a fish bladder, symbol of the floating, of the volatile, as also of the airy, and the atmospheric pressure (it is not a purse, as is sometimes asserted).

The right foot of the old man stands on firm ground, or earth, the left in water. On the Sulfur side we see a king with a solar aura; he is seated on a lion, the zodiacal sign of the sun. Farther below, we can also see a fire-spitting dragon.

On the Mercury side we see Diana with the crescent resting on her head, and the hunting bow. The goddess is riding on a sea monster.

The Salt in the center below stems from the working together of the two Principles Sulfur and Mercury.

All things and beings in the universe contain the three Philosophical Principles. They are the three necessary substances that make the material condensation possible at all.

From the modern viewpoint, we can also call Salt the physical units; Mercury corresponds to undulation; while Sulfur represents the quantum of light. A likewise acceptable analogy would depict the correspondence between proton (Sulfur), electron (Mercury), and neutron (Salt).

In his work *Alchymie und Heilkunst,* Alexander von Bernus designates as "prime matter" negative electricity, which, as a chemical body, is atomistically organized.[21]

In his famous *Book of Hieroglyphic Figures,*[22] Nicolas Flamel says of the relation between Sulfur and Mercury: "these are two snakes that are attached around the caduceus or mercurial staff, by which Mercury derives his great power and transforms himself as desired. . . ." Figure 7 shows the mercurial staff, or caduceus, after a drawing by Hans Holbein the Younger. The two snakes around the staff bestow the power of the *Solve et coagula:* Dissolve and bind. The symbol of the snake-staff appears in many traditions, for instance as the staff of Moses, the staff of Asclepius, the vertebral column entwined with *idā* and *piṅgalā* in yoga representations (figure 8) or as a sculpture or pictorial representation in Indian art (figure 9).

Figure 8 shows the three most important yoga *nāḍīs.* The *nāḍīs* (from the root *nāḍ,* motion) are subtle channels through which flow the vital energies. The coarser channels are the nerves, veins, and arteries, which are also known to Western medicine, while the subtler, through which the *prāṇa* energy flows, have no equivalent counterparts here, just like the meridians of Chinese medicine. The *nāḍīs* with the energy centers (*cakras*) in the central channel, represented in figure 8, are considered the most important *nāḍīs.* They are called *idā, piṅgalā,* and *śuṣumnā.*

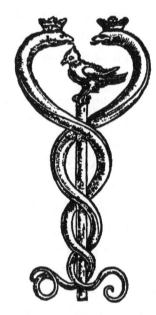

Fig. 7

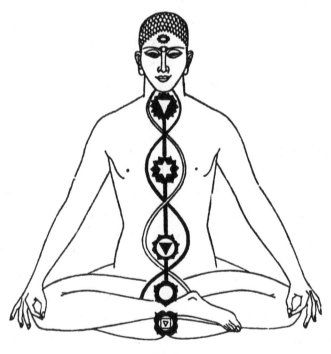

Fig. 8

Here now follows a *synoptical table* of the principal *nāḍīs:*

Name	Iḍā	Śuṣumnā	Piṅgalā
Nature	Moonlike "Embodiment of the nectar"	Fiery	Sunlike
Temperature	Cooling		Heating
Color	Pale	Fiery red	Fiery red
Sex	Female (Śakti-rūpa)		male (Rudra-rūpa)
Course	From the right testicle to the left nostril	In the innermost of the vertebral column	From the left testicle to the right nostril
Corresponding river	Ganges	Sarasvati	Yamuna

The *śuṣumnā* channel unites in itself the moonlike, the sunlike, and the fiery. Within the *śuṣumnā* channel there is the shining *Vajrā-nāḍī* (also called *vajriṇī-nāḍī*), and within the latter flows the pale *citrā* or *cintriṇī- nāḍī,* a moonlike channel whose interior is also called *Brahma-nāḍī.*

Figure 9 represents a Rajasthani miniature painting of the eighteenth century. On an altar we see the *liṅga,* the reproductive organ of god Śiva. On both sides are the snakes that symbolize *iḍā* and *piṅgalā.* The larger, many-headed snake can be recognized as Kundalinī (literally, "the coiled one," i.e., the Serpent Power or Serpent Fire), which rises in the vertebral column (*śuṣumnā*) after its awakening and awakens the *cakras* (see figure 8) one after another. When it reaches the highest *cakra,* the *yogin* simultaneously attains the highest level of consciousness. The altar symbolizes the *yoni,* the female sex organ. The trident with the pennant is a further symbol of Śiva. We can also recognize a bell and various plants, beneath them in the lower right the *tulsī* plant *(Ocimum sanctum),* a variety of basil, which is highly regarded in India. The frame of the pictures is formed by squares of four alchemical colors:

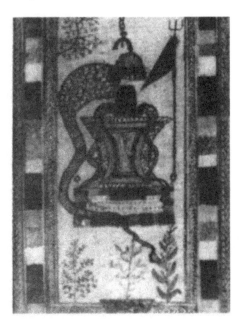

Fig. 9

black, white, red, and gold, which correspond to stages of the Great Work (Nigredo, Albedo, Rubedo, and Projection).

Summarizing, we can say that we observe everywhere in the universe three forces or manifestations simultaneously:

1. The tiny building blocks of the atoms, which form matter—the Salt Principle.
2. The Life Principle, *prāṇa,* which tries to materialize in countless forms, from the simple molecules to the most complicated structures. We recognize in it the Mercury Principle.
3. Consciousness, intelligence, which guides and forms all life. It is the soul, *jīvātman,* or *ātman,* the Sulfur Principle.

In alchemy, the following symbols are used for them:

$$☿ = \text{Mercury}$$
$$🜍 = \text{Sulfur}$$
$$\ominus = \text{Salt}$$

These three Philosophical Principles are accessible to our senses in the form of matter that manifests in four different states: (1) solid, (2) liquid, (3) gaseous, (4) radiant or etheric. These manifestations are considered the four Elements. They are called Earth, Water, Air, and Fire and are endowed with the properties cold, moist, dry, and hot.

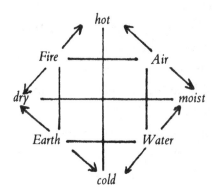

Because of their dual qualities, the Elements can separate and intermingle. In each case, two Elements have one quality in common, and each Element also contains something of the other three. Fire from the Water Element, for instance, would be the product of detonating gas through the separation of hydrogen and oxygen by means of electricity.

The Elements of alchemy are therefore not basic substances in the sense of chemistry but manifest as states of matter. They are represented by the following symbols:

$\triangle$ = Fire
$\triangledown$ = Water
$\triangle$ = Air
$\triangledown$ = Earth

Together they form the symbol ✡, which is also known as Solomon's Seal or the Star of David.

The Element Fire is characterized by the emission of light and heat; the Element Water is the liquid state; the Element Air is gaseous and volatile; and the Element Earth is the concrete, solid condition of matter.

In practical laboratory alchemy, different substances are designated as the Elements, according to the work of the day. In the *Opus Vini,* the *Work of the Wine,* for instance, alcohol is considered Air (because it is volatile); the phlegma remaining after its distillation is Water; the solid residue remaining after the subsequent distillation of the phlegma is Earth; and the shining color of the wine that is distilled by special manual operations is Fire. What matters in the separation of the Elements—which can never be done completely—is to recognize what substances are considered the Elements. The respective alchemistic texts clarify this point each time.

We can reflect still further on the significance of the Elements.

Fire signifies warmth, expansion, the active; furthermore, the creative, the pure, the subtle, the noble, the virtuous, the masculine potency, strength, the will, generosity, altruism, and intuition.

Air, which is denser than Fire, out of which it is precipitated, in the medium between Fire and Water. It is also the "carrier of the seed" and signifies in a broader sense wisdom, clarity, cleanliness, intellect, reason, the ability to communicate, and the expansion of being.

Water is the result of the coagulation of Fire and Air. Steam condenses and turns into water. Water is magnetic and is called "universal menstruum," also "mother of the things." It is either condensed air or liquid earth; its character is cold and contractive. In a broader sense, it signifies the passive, the absorbing, the penetrating, life, feelings, love of nature and of the great family. It acts as a mediator between Air and Earth.

Earth is solid and contains three other Elements in a specially noticeable way. We recognize in it coagulated Fire, coagulated Water, and condensed Air (vapor). It is the mother of metals, minerals, plants, and animals and is therefore also called the Great Treasurer. It is the mother of all material things, which are meant to attain to eternal life through evolution, and through the imperfection of things it provides the knowledge of that which is still lacking for completion.

The alchemist Johannes Isaac Hollandus[23] distinguishes between the two manifested Elements, Water and Earth, and the two inflowing

Elements, Air and Fire. The latter are concealed in the former, Air in Water, and Fire in Earth. Water and Earth are fixed Elements; both are depicted by triangles standing on their points (descending). Fire and Air are volatile; they are represented by upward pointing triangles. In the engraving discussed earlier (figure 9), we see the fixed Elements below; and above, the volatile. The remaining details of the picture refer less to plant alchemy, which is also called the Lesser Work, than to the Great Work, with which we will not deal here.

Within the four Elements a fifth is present, the Quinta Essentia or Quintessence, which is none of the four Elements, however. The Quinta Essentia is considered as permeating the whole of creation. In a way it can be compared to the ether or space (*ākāśa*) of the Indian tradition. "It does everything, and without it nothing can be done," says Raimundus Lullus.[24]

The Quinta Essentia is the force that binds everything, the foundation without which the Elements would be dead matter. It is the spiritual core of all things and, according to Paracelsus, the extract of the Elements, that is, their incorruptible eternal substratum. As such it is simultaneously the origin and the goal of all evolution. The Quinta Essentia is the cohesive force of all living creatures and all existing things. It is also called Mother, Never-Failing Source, Heavenly Water, Universal Spirit, Mercurius, Earth Mother, Mother of the Waters, Ocean, Coelum, Substantia Coelestis, Celestial Menstruum, Radix Substantialis, Apogennēma, Seminarium Mundi, Spiritus Coelesti, and Clavis Philosophorum.

The liberation of the Quinta Essentia, respectively of that which is in each case considered its principal carrier, is characteristic of many spagyric preparations. Thus many magisteria are also called the Quintessence from Wine or the Quintessence of Honey.

In laboratory chemistry various substances are often designated as Quinta Essentia, and a frequently heard theorem says that it is not one of the four Elements but proves to be one of the three Philosophical Principles. In this respect, the designation Quinta Essentia is also used for specific substances, for instance, for ethyl alcohol (spirit of wine) or for the Vegetable Stones, which will be discussed later.

Let us once again visualize a comprehensive diagram:

1. A Divine Principle, which manifests as a union of Prima Materia (primordial matter) and Prima Energia (primordial energy). The two Principles represent a reality and form the foundation of creation (see the picture of Śiva, page 47). The first part of the diagram is occasionally also simply called Prima Materia in alchemy.
2. Polarity or duality: the two Principles Sulfur and Mercury as opposites. In addition, also the opposition between the fixed and the volatile, the *solve* and the *coagula,* Sun and Moon, *yang* and *yin,* and so on. See also figure 10, Hermes Trismegistus with the two Principles and the Fire. "The sun is its father, the moon its mother . . . ," says the Emerald Tablet.[25]
3. The triad or trinity or ternarius: the three Philosophical Principles, meaning the duality Sulfur and Mercury, to which the Principle Salt is added.
4. The quadruplicity or quarternity or quarternarius: the Elements Fire, Water, Air, and Earth.
5. The quintuplicity or set of five: the four forms of manifestation of nature (Elements) with the Quinta Essentia.

In hermetic philosophy nature is considered the totality of all beings in the universe. The totality is animated by the Divine Principle.

In this connection, we will reproduce here a few paragraphs from the address of the *"allerseits geliebten Freunde"* (the everywhere beloved friends) in the compilation *Hermetic ABC.*[26]

§1

True wisdom is the encompassing of all pure truths for the recognition of God outside and inside His creatures, from eternity to eternity, throughout the times determined by Him.

§2

All visible and invisible, countless, various, spiritual and corporeal creatures, so different in their natures, mixtures, species, sizes, powers, properties, destinies, effects, and duration, together with all worlds, live, weave and float in their immeasurable and incomprehensible origin in the inscrutable spirit-being which we call God in our highest understanding.

§3

God carries all His creatures with all the worlds within Himself; He surrounds and fills them all: the heavens, the stars, the sun, the planets, the common air, the whole atmosphere, our seas, water, earth, yes, all individual rational and irrational, living, mobile, growing and resting or seemingly lifeless spiritual and corporeal creatures.

§4

God has in stages engendered, that is, created, out of His own being all His creatures in a wonderful way, incomprehensible to us. He is the origin of all (§2): Out of Him they all have their being and are created.

§5

As He surrounds and fills the heavens, the earth, yes, everything in and upon it (§3), so He sustains all His spiritual as well as material creatures through His constant influence, through His ever-presence; yes, thus He carries all of them within Himself, in His almighty, unlimited, and superperfect spirit-being (§2, §3). He nourishes them like a father and mother, each according to its destination.

§6

This destination has its order, purpose, time, and goal for each of His creatures (§2); from, through, in, and with Him they live, weave, float, are, and remain eternally according to their prime matter.

§7

He causes all their transformations directly or indirectly, in the order of his householding, in and through Himself, at the time determined for each; for the purpose of His wisdom; for His pleasure and for their best in eternity; according to different stages of refining; for the infinite eternal satisfaction, well-being, and destined perfection of each: of which the echo, or their expression and countermovement, will be nothing in the divine order but the glory and praise of their God among and within them, with eternal bliss.

In the beginning, the Divine Principle divides into an active and a passive part: Prima Energia and Prima Materia, called Puruṣa and Prakṛti in Sanskrit, Yang and Yin in the Chinese tradition, Sulfur and Mercury in hermetic philosophy.

The original Mercury is also called Chaotic Water, Abysmal Water, Divine Water, Eternal Water, Silvery Water, Ocean, Great Sea of the Philosophers, Primordial Humidum, Indeterminate Principle of Individuals, Philosophical Basilisk, Feminine Principle.

In its function as opposite of the original energy—the latter is also represented as the dot in the circle (sun symbol)—the original Mercury is also often portrayed as a moon or Diana and is therefore represented by the moon symbol.

The original energy is the Noncreated Fire or the Inner Fire. It is also called the Word of God above the waters, or Dragon's Head, Sun, Original Fire, Original Energy, Formative Principle, Male Principle, or simply Sulfur. Its symbol is the dot in the circle ⊙, manifesting within the Prima Materia ◯. The symbol of the Prima Materia is simultaneously the symbol of the Void, the Nothing, which can give birth to everything.

The Bible describes this process in the following words (Genesis 1:2–4):

And the earth was without form and void: and darkness was upon the face of the deep. And the Spirit of God moved upon the face

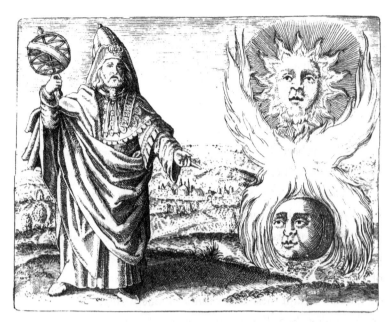

Fig. 10

of the waters [= Prima Materia = ◯]. And God said, Let there be light: and there was light.

(Light is born within darkness. The two Principles are here still forming a unit. This will become clear as we read on):

And God saw the light, that it was good; and God divided the light from the darkness. . . .

In this way the polarity between the Principles arises:

• and ◯

Yang and Yin

♀ and ☿

Finally, on the second and third day of creation, the solid, the "Salt," also appears, and on the fourth day of creation, the Sun and Moon. We must not mistake the original light of the first day of creation for the Sun and Moon of the fourth day.

Let us now listen to Johannes Isaac Hollandus. In his work *Opera Vegetabilia* he writes about Creation:[27]

> Therefore, let my child be aware that the first matter of everything in the world has been ☿; since water existed before there was even time, and the Spirit of the Lord rested on it. But what kind of water was it? Was it cloudwater? Or another kind that one could pour? No, but it was a dry, slimy water into which God set His earth, which was His Sulfur, so that the earth coagulated the water, and there arose from it the four Elements which had been locked in these two by command of God and His supreme Will. ☿ dissolves the Sulfur, and Sulfur coagulates ☿, and these two cannot be one without the other. ☿ is never without the Sulfur because it is transformed into it. The nature proper of ☿ is that it dissolves its Sulfur and makes it white, and the nature of the dry Sulfur purges and congeals its ☿. As these two cannot be one without the other, they also cannot be without Salt. The latter is the principal means whereby Nature accomplishes her generation of all things in the whole world, in vegetables, minerals, as well as in animals, which teaching of mine you should well understand. For if Nature did not have ☿ in her generation straight at the beginning of the original composition of every created thing, the latter could not keep together in its natural moisture, which is one of the most necessary ingredients for keeping a thing in its essence. And if she did not have the Sulfur, the moist parts would not be congealed. Likewise if she did not have the Salt (which is the means whereby she connects both and causes one to enter the other), it would neither mingle with anything in the world nor unite with it, because there would be no sharpness for entering, and it could not unite with anything. Consequently, these three, namely ☿, 🜍, and ⊖, are none without the other; where you find one of them, you find them all three, and there is no created thing in the world wherein you do not find them. From these three everything has arisen that is in the world.

They are also so much intermixed in the four Elements that they are one in one body. The Salt, however, is hiding in the deepest part of the Elements because it must keep them together by its sharpness and dryness. It is nevertheless a spirit and volatile. However, because it is contained in the deepest of the mixture and is kept captive by the fat-combustible oil to which it clings—for the Salt is contained in the combustible oil like the yolk in the egg, and the combustible oil lies in the deepest part of the Elements where it separates last from the Earth together with the Salt and fecibus—the Salt lies buried at the bottom of the Earth and the combustible oil. Consequently, it cannot flee from the Earth except by the power of the Fire, or else the three aforementioned spirits must first separate from the mixture of the Elements, which is the soul of all things or their Qu.Ess., which must keep the whole mixture of the Elements together, and when it is extracted, this mixture separates of its own. Thereafter the Salt must not be separated from the Earth with the Fire, but when all the Elements separate from the fecibus, the Salt also separates. This Salt is an unknown Salt to the ignorant, because it is contained in the deepest of the Elements. Therefore, all those who do not know this Salt must necessarily be mistaken, because without this Salt no thing on earth can stay together or come together.

To round off the aforesaid, here is an excerpt from Georg von Welling's work *Opus Mago-Cabbalisticum et Theosophicum:*[28]

§5. Moses teaches us in chapter 1 of Genesis, when he describes the creation of the whole world, or of our solar system, that the Almighty God created in the beginning *shamayim v'et haarets,* that is, the heavens or primeval waters, and the earth. Here Moses puts the heavens, the spiritual fiery water, first, and he does so not without a very special reason; for they are the beginning of all things first created by the Lord God, or the beginning of beginnings, which is almost unfathomable for us in its true nature, as its wondrous name lets us sufficiently recognize; for Moses, or rather the Holy Ghost through Moses, calls this extension *shamayim,* which is a composite name that has been described by the rabbinical elders, who were trained and experienced in the true Kabbalah, as being composed of *esh* and *mayim,* fire and water. This is in truth, according to the outer letter, a very wonderful and strange mixture, and how is it possible to mix two such quite opposite things so harmoniously? Which, however, is an eternal truth; only that this fiery water, or watery fire, without which no creature can live and be maintained, is sought by so few in order to know it. To describe it in its whole sphaera is just not our purpose; besides, a more experienced pen is probably required for such Divine Secrets as ours. . . .

Finally, a look at the Indian conceptual world.

In the Indian and Tibetan tradition, the dot (*bindu*) represents consciousness (see figure 11).

The nasal character of the *mantras* in Sanskrit is indicated by the sign ◡ over a vocal or a consonant.

For instance:

$$\pi = ga, \quad \smile = m\dot{m} = a\dot{m} \text{ (nasal)}, \quad \overset{\smile}{\pi} = gam^{29}$$

The sign ◡ is literally called *candrabindu* (moon and dot). All *bija mantras* (seed syllables)[30] contain these two principles, about which we have already heard.

Primordial energy is indestructible, but when it combines with matter and goes with it through the stage of decaying, which separates the pure from the impure, it stimulates the purified components to a new materialization.

With every decaying *(putrefactio)* the matter is exalted. Thus, out of the bodies of the mineral kingdom arise those of the plant world, and out of the latter those of the animal world.

This cosmic process of evolution, of creation and destruction to make room again for a new creation, has found its perfect portrayal in the figure of the Indian Naṭarāja, the Lord of the Dance (see illustration below). The god Śiva, as Lord of the Dance, represents the dynamic cosmic processes.

Śiva's right side is male, the left female. Both together form one single being. One of the god's names is Svayambhū, the Self-existent.

In one of his right hands we see the *ḍamarū,* a double drum shaped like an hourglass. With this drum he initiates creation by creating time and its periods. In one of his left hands he is holding the fire that not only animates the created but also destroys it, so that a new creation can follow. By fire, matter is purified and exalted.

With his other right hand he blesses his creation with a protective gesture. With his other left hand he points to his raised foot, which symbolizes salvation.

His right foot is standing on a recumbent dwarf, who symbolizes the forces of evil, which the divine dancer dominates and controls.

In Naṭarāja's hair, which swings in the air, we see the moon and the river Ganges (Water).

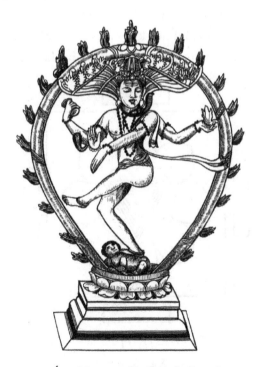

Śiva Naṭarāja (Lord of the Dance)

The stage of the dance is the cosmic space *(ākāśa),* indicated by a crown of cosmic fire.

In figure 11, the circle represents ignorance *(avidyā).* The eight leaves of the lotus form the aspects of Prakṛti; Earth, Water, Fire, Air, Ether, mind *(mānas),* intellect *(buddhi),* and egoism *(ahaṁkāra).*

The five triangles are the five *Jñānendriyas (jñāna,* wisdom; *indriyas,* the senses); the five *karmendriyas* (organs of action), and the five kinds of *prāṇa* (vital force); the dot *(bindu)* in the center is pure consciousness.

Underneath the whole we see as ashlar, or square stone, the earth or matter that carries the sculpture.

In this way, all the Elements are represented.

Upon all this, dear reader, you should reflect deeply. Bear ever in mind that the names Fire, Water, Air, Earth, Mercury, Sulfur, and so on, must never be mistaken for their usual meaning. Then some views that are still held today by historians of chemistry—for instance, that alchemists took all metals to be mercuric sulfates—will be corrected on their own.

The masters of old of course had no conceptions in line with modern scientific chemistry. They did not know, for example, that calcined tartar (or hydrogen potassium tartrate) consists in the main of potassium

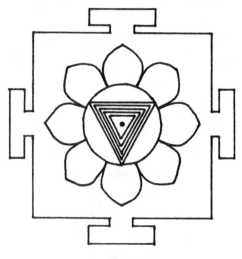

Fig. 11
Kālī Yantra

carbonate. The concept of potassium carbonate did not exist at all. Potassium carbonate can be produced in different ways, for instance, by the sublimation of degreased wool or by the calcination of plants and the subsequent extraction of the salt. The chemical formula is the same. The alchemists did not know this, and it would have been of little interest to them from the point of view of their art. Much more important to them was the possibility of making the calcined tartar volatile. They knew how to distill it to cure certain diseases with the distillate. With it, for instance, they could dissolve uric acid in the body and expel it. The distillation of potassium carbonate, like that of alkaline salts in general, is impossible, however, in the opinion of scientific chemistry. In the volatilization of tartar, it is therefore a question of a change in chemical composition. It is indeed so, and regarding this misunderstanding, which caused the German alchemist Alexander von Bernus to lose a lawsuit, the difference between the chemical and the alchemical conception regarding this case will now be briefly described.

Intermezzo:
The Volatilization of Tartar

Tartar is the salt of tartaric acid. Tartaric acid occurs naturally and also as both calcium salt and potash salt in fruit, hence also in grapes. Since tartaric acid has two asymmetrical carbon atoms, we can find it in three different forms:

COOH	COOH	COOH
H—C—OH	HO—C—H	H—C—OH
HO—C—H	H—C—OH	H—C—H
COOH	COOH	COOH
= *dextrorotatory* *(turning to the right)* *tartaric acid*	= *levorotatory* *(turning to the left)* *tartaric acid*	= *mesotartaric acid* *(optically inactive)*

Substances that distort the plane of polarized light in the positive angle are called dextrorotatory; levorotatory means the reverse. A mixture of the same number of molecules of both forms neutralizes the effect of both and is therefore called optically inactive. All three forms of tartaric acid have the same number of atoms; only the position of the two central groups—OH—is different.

Only the dextrorotatory tartaric acid is found uncombined in nature. It can form two different potassium salts by replacing one or two hydrogen atoms by a potassium atom.

In the first instance we have the replacement of a hydrogen atom by a potassium atom:

$$
\begin{array}{c}
\mathrm{C-OOK} \\
| \\
\mathrm{H-C-OH} \\
| \\
\mathrm{HO-C-H} \\
| \\
\mathrm{C-OOH}
\end{array}
$$

This is potassium bitartrate or acid tartrate, which is dextrorotatory. In the second instance, we have the replacement of two hydrogen atoms by two potassium atoms:

$$
\begin{array}{c}
\mathrm{C-OOK} \\
| \\
\mathrm{H-C-OH} \\
| \\
\mathrm{HO-C-H} \\
| \\
\mathrm{C-OOK}
\end{array}
$$

This structural formula can be recognized as potassium tartrate. It is neutral and also dextrorotatory.

Only the first-mentioned of these two salts occurs abundantly on the walls of the containers in which the must is fermented into wine. In alchemy, this salt is called Tartarus Crudus (crude tartar). In addition to acid tartrate, Tartarus Crudus also contains calcium tartrate.

By a treatment with fire (heat), coal, and clay (the alchemical masters recommend the powder of tiles) as well as other methods, Tartarus Crudus can be "purified." The result is Tartarus Depuratus (purified tartar), also called Cremor Tartari (cream of tartar), which contains no more calcium tartrate. We are in fact now dealing with approximately 99 percent of acid tartrate. This is insoluble but can be partly dissolved in boiling water; in twenty parts of water one part of tartrate can be dissolved.

If the Tartarus Depuratus is calcined, it forms a black coal-like mass. (Because of the strong formation of smoke, the calcination had better be done under a hood or in the open air.)

This calcined tartar is now no longer acid tartar but is alkaline and hygroscopic. By dissolving it in water with subsequent filtration and evaporation of the water, we can make the salt visible. Chemically viewed, this substance can no longer be called tartar. For the chemist, however, the result is Tartarus Depuratus Calcinatus (purified calcined tartar), although the chemist rightly asserts from the vantage of his science that this substance may well have been made from tartar but no longer has anything in common with the original tartar.

Now let us take yet another step forward.

This substance is transformed once again through volatilization.

Different ways exist to achieve this, among them cohobation with rectified wine vinegar, which is frequently mentioned in alchemistic treatises.[31] But there are still various other ways.

In the opinion of chemists, the original tartar is thus constantly transformed into other substances. But only the original substance, to which we have finally "lent wings" by our various treatments, deserves the name *tartar* within the meaning of chemistry, and it is not volatile. As far as the rest is concerned, it is a question of other substances for the chemist.

Of course the chemist is right from the viewpoint of his science. For the alchemist, on the other hand, tartar appears in four different forms: as Tartarus Crudus, as Tartarus Depuratus, as Tartarus Depuratus Calcinatus, and as "volatile tartar." The confusion is due to linguistic usage and related concepts.

Such examples are frequent in alchemy. The controversy about whether or not it is possible to extract the tincture out of antimony by means of rectified vinegar also belongs here. Many alchemists have worked the corresponding processes after the pattern of those described in the *Triumphal Chariot of Antimony* of Basilius Valentinus. Strictly speaking, it is a question of tinctures made with the help of antimony, because antimony here acts as a catalyst. An American spagyric producer therefore rightly calls his corresponding product "triacetic antimonious catalysate." But this by no means signifies that the "antimony tinctures" (or tinctures from or by antimony) do not contain the curative powers of antimony.

True alchemy is not at variance with scientific chemistry if it is rightly understood. It is a matter of two different planes of understanding and working.

An engineer who is building a hydroelectric plant is chiefly interested in water power, that is, in the utilization of the force of gravity as it acts upon the water, because it is this that drives his turbines. The gardener, in contrast, will be more interested in the vital power of the water. We must not confuse the planes.

What did Basilius say in his "five points"?: "fourth: the applications; and fifth: the usefulness. . . ." We should reflect on this.

After we have dealt somewhat with the world of conceptions and the theoretical foundations, we shall turn to the practice in the following chapters.

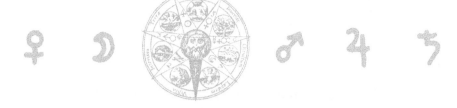

4

MERCURY, SULFUR, AND SALT IN THE PLANT WORLD

In all three realms—the mineral, plant, and animal worlds—Mercury is always a volatile substance on the material plane, Sulfur an oily substance, and Salt a substance of solid consistency. More precisely, we would have to say: the carriers of the Mercury Principle, the Sulfur Principle, and the Salt Principle. Mercury itself (spirit) is intangible. The relation is so close, however, that the carrier of the Mercury Principle is simply called Mercury in laboratory chemistry, likewise the corresponding substances as Sulfur, respectively Salt.

In the plant world, ethyl alcohol (ethanol = C_2H_5OH) is the carrier of the Mercury Principle. In some treatises, ethyl alcohol is also designated as the Element Air, or even as the Quinta Essentia, but those are exceptions that should not confuse the reader. In a narrower sense, we always consider ethyl alcohol the Mercury of the plant world.

Ethyl alcohol is not found in free form in nature, but it can be extracted from plants by fermentation and subsequent distillation.

During fermentation, the plant is decomposed, and the grape sugar contained in it, to which the Mercury Principle is bound (a monosaccharide, $C_6H_{12}O_6$), is changed into ethyl alcohol and carbon monodixe after the formula:

$$C_6H_{12}O_6 \mapsto 2\ C_2H_5OH + 2\ CO_2$$

Fermentation occurs through yeasts, living microorganisms that produce a ferment called zymase. It converts the sugar into alcohol and carbon dioxide.

We can also obtain alcohol from the polysaccharides cellulose and starch by decomposing them. Both consist of grape sugar molecules, but we cannot replace cellulose and starch directly by yeasts.

Here now are the structures of cellulose, starch, and grape sugar:

cellulose

starch

grape sugar

There are different kinds of yeast. The kinds that are of interest to us here are brewer's yeast and wine yeast. The degree of activity of the yeasts depends on the temperature of the surroundings. The most favorable temperature for the fermentation of wine yeast is approximately 20–25° C.

During fermentation, the so-called fusel oils are also formed. They consist of other alcohols and waste products of proteins. As they are not part of Mercury, they must be removed in the distillation of the alcohol. During fermentation, the alcohol content rises slowly. When it has reached about 15 percent, the activity of the yeasts is checked, and it finally stops altogether. A prerequisite is that the solution to be fermented contain a sufficiently large quantity of grape sugar to attain such a high percentage; otherwise the attainable quantity of alcohol will stay far below the figure just mentioned. This is also the case in the fermentation of plants without the addition of completely fermentable kinds of sugar. When the fermentation is finished, the alcohol is distilled off and subsequently rectified. More about that later.

It is important to remember that the Mercury Principle is always anonymous and therefore does not appear to be bound to the individual plant species. Throughout the whole plant world, ethyl alcohol is the carrier of Mercury, while Sulfur and Salt belong exclusively to the respective species. We can therefore replace Mercury in the plant world at any time "from outside," thus, for instance, also buy it in the drugstore. And we can then safely use this ethyl alcohol as Mercury in all spagyric preparations from plants, since it is not proper to the species. This basic knowledge also explains why some spagyrists add completely fermentable sugars to their plant ingredients to be fermented. The anonymous character of Mercury permits this manipulation as long as Mercury is only extracted from substances of *plant* origin, because in the plant world Mercury is always the same. We should nevertheless not overlook the fact that ethyl alcohol is considered the noblest and best carrier of Mercury and therefore plays a special role in plant alchemy. The reason lies in the substances and energies that are bound up with the ethyl alcohol of the wine. For this reason the origin plays a role nevertheless. After all, there is Mercury and Mercury, just as there is water and water. Besides, it is almost impossible to get completely pure ethyl alcohol. So-called absolute alcohol also contains small amounts of other substances.

Ethyl alcohol is an easily combustible, clear, colorless liquid, simultaneously fire, water, and air.

Sulfur appears in a double form in the plant world, as volatile and as fixed Sulfur.

The etheric or essential oils of the plants represent volatile Sulfur. We obtain fixed Sulfur by evaporating the fermented liquid, after previously distilling off Mercury (ethyl alcohol) and volatile Sulfur (the etheric oils), and after the solid components of the plant residue have been removed by filtration.

The liquid is repeatedly evaporated until there remains a tarlike or honeylike mass that during the evaporation almost reminds one of lava. This "honey" is the fixed Sulfur. Accordingly, plants without essential oils also possess their Sulfur.

If we continue with the evaporation of fixed Sulfur, it finally forms a hard black mass. If we heat it still more, it changes gradually into a gray or grayish-white ash. The salts contained in this ash are the salt of the Sulfur, to which we shall return later. The essential oils, the volatile Sulfur, are complex mixtures of many substances. Whereas Mercury is the same in the whole plant world, the composition of the etheric oils varies strongly from plant to plant. It is precisely this Sulfur that gives every plant its special individuality. The Sulfur is always that which is truly individual, the soul, its essence. This is the reason why these oils are called essential oils. An entire therapeutic system, aromatherapy, is based exclusively on the application of essential oils and their curative powers. The content of essential oils in plants fluctuates very much with environmental factors. With an appropriate neighborhood for the plants, for instance in stinging nettles, it can be considerably increased, up to 20 percent in valerian, over 80 percent in angelica, 10 to 20 percent in marjoram, and 10 percent in sage and peppermint.[32]

Essential oils are liquid at room temperature, burn with a sooting flame, do not mix with water but float on top of it, and are volatile. We are dealing with strongly aromatic substances that show a strong kinship with heat (fire) elements. The essential oil of rosemary, for instance, is the compound richest in hydrogen in the plant world, and hydrogen is the substance most akin to heat in the universe. The vapor of the essential oils is colorless and transparent. It allows light to pass through practically without hindrance, and while it absorbs the heat rays of the light, the light from the vapor is cold. Such a behavior is called diathermy.

Steam distillation is the best method for the extraction of essential oils from plants. In the next chapter we will familiarize ourselves with this technique.

If Mercury is the spirit and Sulfur the soul, Salt is the "body" of the plants. It is neither volatile nor liquid but is the only one of the Philosophical Principles that is solid and incombustible.

The salt of the plants can be made visible through incineration and subsequent calcination (literally, making white) of the plants or the plant residues respectively.

Basilius describes the production of plant salts as follows:

How the Salia can be extracted from all herbs and plants. Take whatever herb you wish, burn it to ashes, make a lye of it with warm water, coagulate the lye, then the salt will stay in fundo, resolve it in Spiritu Vini. Throw away the Feces that will settle, draw off the Spiritum Vinum per Destillationem, and resolve it frequently until the salt is beautifully clear and pure and leaves no more Feces; then it is ready. If one proceeds with the purification of the Spiritus Vini in the right way, all the salts of herbs can be made beautiful, clean, and pure, so that they sprout transparently into crystals, like a clean, purified saltpeter.[33]

Salt prepared in this way contains the "body" and also the salt of the fixed Sulfur. From this preparation neither Mercury nor Sulfur can be obtained, since they must be extracted before calcination. But we may well prepare the salt from the plant residue after the separation of Sulfur and Mercury from the plant residue. To not confuse the salt of Sulfur (part of the soul) with the "body," the former is also called Sal Sulfuris (Salt of the Sulfur) and the latter, Sal Salis (Salt of the Salt).

Each of the two salts can be divided into two substances. One part is water-soluble, the other is not.

The extraction of the water-soluble salts is done as follows:

The calcined ash is put in a beaker and covered with double or triple the amount of distilled water. Everything is slowly heated and stirred. Now the water-soluble salts dissolve, while the insoluble ones settle. The clear liquid is decanted and filtered.

To extract the water-soluble salts without residue, the process must be repeated several times, until litmus paper no longer shows a higher pH-value than that of the distilled water used. Finally, the salt solution is carefully evaporated at low temperatures (for instance, in the sun), and the white salts stay behind. During the evaporation, the temperature must be kept low or else the salt solution sputters violently.

Should the solution of the salts in distilled water show an orange-colored streak, the calcination of the plant residues was insufficient. The proper execution of calcination is one of the most difficult kinds of manual work in alchemy. We shall return to it later in detail. If the first calcination was not sufficient, the evaporated salt must once again be calcined. Thereafter, it is again dissolved in distilled water, the solution is filtered anew, and the water again evaporated until the salt is dry. Since the salt is strongly hygroscopic, it is kept in sealed, airtight glass containers. Water-soluble salts are always alkaline.

The residue that remains after filtration of the solution is also called Caput Mortuum (Death's Head). To get the Caput Mortuum quite pure, we must rinse it many times with distilled water. The pH-factor can be tested with litmus paper. Chemically viewed, the water-soluble salts consist chiefly of potassium carbonate and approximately 10 to 20 percent of other salts, such as potassium chloride, potassium sulfate, and sodium carbonate. The salts are fusible at about 900°. The salts that are not water-soluble (Caput Mortuum) consist chiefly of calcium, silicon, phosphorus, and magnesium. They also contain traces of other metals. To melt the Caput Mortuum, temperatures of over 1500° are required.

The Caput Mortuum is not hygroscopic and amorphous, while the soluble salts, if sufficiently pure, form beautiful crystals, especially if they are further purified by repeated dissolving in distilled water with subsequent filtration and evaporation of the solution.

5

THE EXTRACTION OF THE THREE PHILOSOPHICAL PRINCIPLES FROM PLANTS

The separation of a plant into the three Philosophical Principles or Essentials always begins with the extraction of the essential oils, which represent the volatile part of the Sulfur.

The reason is that the essential oils are soluble in alcohol. If we let the plant go through fermentation to obtain Mercury (ethyl alcohol), the latter will indeed also extract the essential oils in the process of formation *(in statu nascendi),* but the bond between Sulfur (essential oils) and Mercury (ethyl alcohol) is so strong in this instance that they can hardly ever be completely separated from each other again. Even the most complicated fractionating techniques, including the freezing process, fractionating columns, centrifuging, or chemical techniques, would never lead to a complete separation, at least not in the alchemical sense.

Another question is whether the separation of Sulfur and Mercury, that is, of the essential oils and ethyl alcohol, is necessary or desirable in all cases of spagyric separation. As it is, alcohol *in statu nascendi* (when forming during fermentation) extracts the essential oils from a plant in a particularly gentle way and then carries them over during a subsequent distillation. If we wish to disengage this "Sulfuric Mercury," we do not need to distill the essential oils before fermentation. We shall see later, when discussing various methods of preparation in detail, that the distilling of the "Sulfuric Mercury" is used in several instances. This kind of distillation must be performed with a certain expertness, if a large part of the volatile Sulfur is not to be lost.

But as we are for the moment dealing with the separation of a plant into all three Principles or Essentials, we must begin with the extraction of the volatile Sulfur, the soul, that is, the essential oils. We understand why the classical directions refer to it again and again. "In the first place, however, you must always extract the soul. . . ." "Let your Sulfur first of all fly out, and catch it well. . . ." "After Apollo has appeared . . . ,"[34] that is, after the essential oils (Sulfur, soul-Apollo) have been distilled off. Thus and similarly are the directions always worded.

Let us therefore begin in this way.

The Extraction of the Essential Oils, That Is, of the Volatile Sulfur

A large number of medicinal plants contain a considerable amount of essential oils. Especially rich in volatile Sulfur is the family of the labiates (Labiatae). In this family, comprising about three thousand species, which directly represents the prototype of the family of medicinal plants—all its species are medicinal—we find our known favorites: rosemary, the mints, basil, balm, which are everywhere easily available. If we cultivate these plants in our own garden, we can considerably increase their content in volatile Sulfur by giving them a proper neighborhood of other plants, for example, by planting them together with stinging nettles.

Rosemary and peppermint are rich in essential oils; we shall appropriately begin with one of these plants. Later we shall come back to species of plants that have little or no volatile Sulfur.

There exist a number of different methods for the extraction of essential oils from plants. The method of enfleurage, known especially in the manufacture of perfume, consists in pressing plants on paraffin plates. The essential oils go over into the fat, out of which they can then be dissolved with alcohol. This method is of less interest to us here.

For our laboratory work the following techniques are suitable:

A. Boiling of the plants in water with simultaneous distillation of the steam and the oils that are then swimming on the water
B. Distillation by means of steam
C. Extraction with a so-called oil separator, without doubt the most elegant and best method

We shall briefly describe all three methods.

Distillation by Boiling in Water

Distillation is a technique whereby volatile substances can be separated from nonvolatile (fixed) ones, or also different liquids from each other in case they have different high boiling points. In the last instance we speak of fractionating.

In the case of a dry distillation, volatile constituents are extracted from solid substances by heat. As examples we would cite the distillation of coal or wood and also of wool.

In some cases the distillate is of greater interest, in others the residue. During the distillation of liquids, the latter are converted by boiling into vapors, which are then changed back into their liquid state in a condenser (cooler) through which flows cooling water, to be collected again as distillate in a collecting vessel, the receiver or receptacle.

The classical masters of alchemy distinguish between various kinds of distillation, several of which will be discussed in section 2 of this chapter. We reduce our plants to small pieces, put them into a sufficiently large glass flask, and add water until about one-third or half of the flask is filled with it. If we use dry plants, we let them soak at least one day. In the case of fresh plants, we can immediately begin with the extraction. We connect the flask with a condenser above a fractionating column, for instance a Liebig condenser, at the other end of which we attach the receptacle to a receiver adapter with an opening to equalize the pressure (figure 12).

Distillation heads that can be provided with a thermometer are practical, as this can show us the boiling point. Particularly in the separation of liquids, exact adherence to the temperatures is important. All appliances are fastened to a stand with practical clamps for stability.

As heating sources, gas burners, hot plates (in the case of flasks with a flat bottom), or the practical electric mantle are suitable.

Whoever seriously considers the installation of a laboratory should consider the acquisition of an electric mantle. It permits the use of thick-walled, round-bottomed flasks, which are also suitable for distillation under vacuum. The electric mantles are often provided with thermostatic controls that make possible the exact regulation of temperatures. In addition, some models have practical support columns. While not a necessity, they certainly simplify alchemical work.

A water bath, an oil bath, or a sand bath is also practical.

On a heating plate we heat a pot with water, oil, or sand (according to the requirements of the temperatures), into which the flask is plunged halfway. We can regulate the heat of the heating plate quite exactly, especially if it has a thermostatic control. Laboratory baths are also available through equipment dealers, but they are relatively expensive.

When assembling the glass appliances, we always put some vacuum

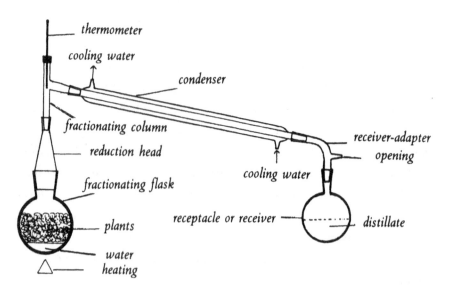

Fig. 12

grease on the glass joints. It not only guarantees their tight closing but also facilitates the later disassembling of the appliances.

When our equipment is assembled (figure 12), we let cooling water flow slowly through the condenser and commence heating up to the boiling point. The rising steam now mounts into the condenser, where it condenses again, finally to run into the receiver as distillate. In so doing, the steam takes along the essential oils, which now float on the surface of the water.

When we have distilled over enough liquid (please do not let the herbs burn!), we put the distillate into a separator (figure 13) and draw the water off below through the drain. We collect the oil that follows in a small, tightly closing bottle. If the oil has not yet all come out of the plants, we pour the remaining water back into the fractionating flask and distill once more; we repeat this until no more oil appears. The process is slow and complicated, but in this way we can carry out the extraction of the volatile Sulfur with simple equipment.

A good specialty store for laboratory equipment will gladly assemble the appliances required in each case. It is advisable to decide on a joint size code, for instance 29/32, to make sure that all appliances are well matched without needing reduction heads or adapters.

Before every experiment, we should mentally go over all details, making sure that everything necessary is at hand, so that we do not make

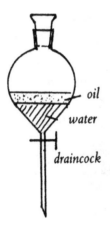

Fig. 13

any mistakes. We can only heat if the possibility of pressure compensation has been taken care of (the receiver-adapter must have an opening), otherwise the distillation will end up on the ceiling!

For plant distillations, flasks with a wide neck are very practical, as they facilitate the later removal of the residue. Of course, they necessitate the use of a reduction column.

Distillation by Means of Steam

We generate steam in a round or Erlenmeyer flask. Through a bent glass or a plastic hose we lead the steam into a flask with two necks that contains the chopped-up plants. Perforated rubber stoppers take care of the sealing. With this flask we then connect, as before, the distilling head, the condenser, the receiver-adapter, and the receptacle (figure 14).

If so-called wide-necked reaction vessels are at our disposal, we can keep the plants above the water level by an inserted sieve (figure 15). Another possibility is the use of an Aludel flask (figure 16), in whose lower neck a narrow glass spiral or a small filter is inserted. The lower flask contains the water.

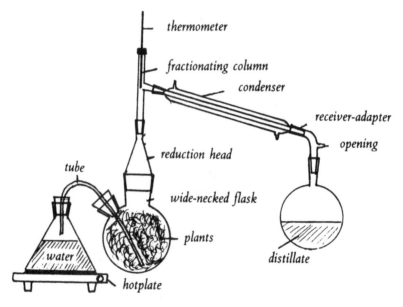

Fig. 14

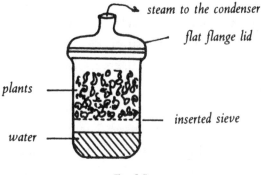

steam to the condenser

flat flange lid

plants

inserted sieve

water

Fig. 15

Whoever intends to work regularly at the distillation of larger quantities of essential oils should consider converting a large stainless steel pressure cooker. Instead of the valve, a corresponding connection is inserted with which we can connect our glass equipment. A perforated rubber stopper, which we can easily replace after use, is enough. The heating can be done with a hot plate.

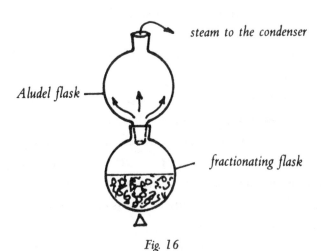

steam to the condenser

Aludel flask

fractionating flask

Fig. 16

Distillation with an Oil Separator

The basic arrangement is the same as already discussed, that is, either the cooking equipment or that for steam distillation. Instead of the distilling head, we put on a so-called oil separator, upon which the condenser is mounted. Especially suitable is a coil condenser, several models of which are available. We can either put on a large condenser (expensive!) or two smaller ones with the aid of a distribution column (U-tube). The condenser stays open above (figure 17), controlled by a stopcock or pinch clamp on flexible tubing.

The steam that carries the essential oils along reaches the condenser through tube A, where it is condensed. The two liquids, oil and water, now drip into tube B. Essential oil is lighter than water and floats on top. Gradually the surface of the liquid rises parallel in tubes E and B. When the liquid reaches point C, the reflux of the water into the fractionating flask begins, while the amount of oil in tube B increases continuously.

The equipment can work for a prolonged period without supervision once the temperature is regulated to a fixed position. There is no danger of burning, as the water flows back continuously.

If the expected amount of oil is quite large, we draw the oil off from time to time through drain D, or else part of the oil might flow back over point C. For this reason some oil separators have a convexly enlarged tube B (dotted line).

When the amount of oil no longer increases, we turn the heating and water cooling off.

If, after reaching the boiling point, our heating and cooling are regulated to a fixed position, we can close the condenser on top. In this way the entire circulation is hermetically sealed off and nothing can get into the equipment. We must, however, pay attention to the precise temperature regulation. Immediately after turning off the heating, the stopper is to be removed so that the pressure compensation can take place during the cooling of the installation.

Let us remember once again that we can immediately extract the oils from fresh plants, whereas dry plants must be macerated for one or several days. Glauber recommends up to three or four days of maceration.[34] But in no case must the plants go through fermentation. Beware of summer temperatures!

Even more ingenious is the drawing off of the essential oils under

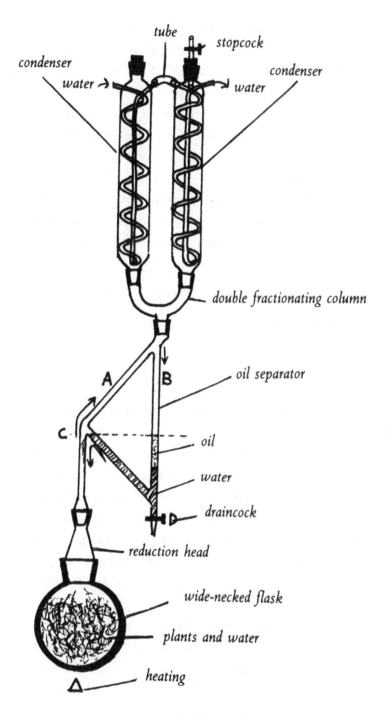

tube

stopcock

condenser

water →

water

condenser

A

B

oil separator

C

oil

water

D   draincock

double fractionating column

reduction head

wide-necked flask

plants and water

heating

Fig. 17

vacuum. A vacuum is made over the upper opening of the condenser by means of a proper pump. The boiling point is thereby greatly reduced, and the drawing off of the essential oils takes place in a specially gentle way (that is, less heat is required). We make use of such an installation when the essential oils contain alkaloids (e.g., in distilling valerian), since alkaloids are sensitive to high temperatures and lose their effectiveness. With valerian, for instance, we must not go over 82° C. Lower temperatures are even better.

We make sure in advance that our equipment is suitable for vacuum distillation, otherwise an explosion might result. Such a danger cannot be altogether excluded, so we protect our eyes with safety goggles.

Mercury

The production of Mercury results from the separation and the subsequent rectification.

Separation

After the drawing off of the essential oils, the remaining plant "soup" is subjected to fermentation.

Everything is put into a sufficiently large glass flask (the formation of foam is to be expected), and an adequate amount of brewer's yeast or dregs of wine is added—that is, 25 grams for 5 quarts of soup.

On the flask we put a cork with a small fermentation tube and some water or oil (figure 18). If we cannot obtain a sufficiently large flask or carboy, we can also ferment in a large preserving jar or a glazed earthenware container. We then close the container by laying a cloth loosely over it and putting a plate on top.

At room temperature fermentation now starts quickly.

Sooner or later fermentation would also occur without any addition of yeast, especially in an open container. This is because the necessary microorganisms are nearly everywhere. Owing to the previous boiling, our plant soup is sterile, however, and therefore the addition of yeast induces more rapid fermentation. Simultaneously, sterility protects our

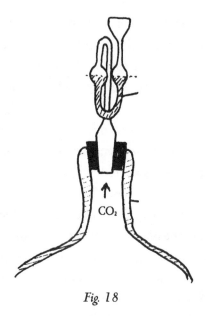

Fig. 18

soup from foreign yeasts and bacteria, whereby we avoid a possible sudden change of the fermentation characteristics.

There exist different ways of fermentation, fermentation combined with lactic acid, acetic fermentation, butyric fermentation, and so on. We are here interested only in alcoholic fermentation, and that is why a stopper with a small fermentation tube is especially advisable. Penetration by other organisms is thus excluded, and a sudden change in the fermentation process need not be feared.

To nourish the yeasts and to reach a specially lively fermentation and a high alcoholic content, we can add a certain amount of fermentable sugar (up to 1 kilogram for 5 quarts of soup) since some plants contain very little sugar. This technique is permitted since Mercury is the same in the whole plant world.[35] Of course, it should always be quite pure. If we intend to obtain but small quantities of Mercury, we can by all means ferment without sugar. But to do this, large quantities of plants are necessary. Glauber recommends at least 50 pounds.[36]

The duration of the fermentation varies greatly from plant to plant, and the temperature also plays a role. It is done when the gas production stops and the plants sink to the bottom.

In the fermentation container we find the four Elements. The plants together with the sugar are the Element Earth. The Element Water is also present. The Element Air is released in the form of gas (carbon dioxide). The Element Fire can be recognized by the liberation of heat energy during fermentation.

In the midst of these four Elements alcohol develops, which, however, is not identical with any of the Elements. This is our Mercury, which is therefore sometimes also designated as Quinta Essentia. An often-heard alchemical theorem is: The Quinta Essentia is none of the Four [Elements] but proves to be one of the Three [Philosophical Principles].

The sugar (that in the plants as well as that which is added), the solid or the fixed, becomes volatile (gas development); the life principle, on the contrary, becomes fixed by condensing into alcohol. Hence also the designation Aqua Vitae (water of life).

We must now distill off and concentrate (rectify) the alcohol that has arisen through fermentation, whereby it is cleansed of its excess water.

Purification

By means of distillation we can separate the liquids from solid substances and likewise liquids with different boiling points from each other. The boiling point is that temperature at which a substance changes from the liquid to the gaseous state.

If we wish to separate two liquids with different boiling points, constant adherence to the boiling-point temperature of the lower-boiling liquid is sufficient. In this way only one of the two liquids can evaporate while the other remains in the fractionating flask, at least for the major part. Part of the higher-boiling liquid, however, is swept along in the evaporation of the lower-boiling one. The separation of the two liquids must therefore be repeated several times. The more strictly we keep to the temperature, the more successful the separation will be.

We begin the purification of Mercury with the separation of the plant soup into a solid and a liquid part by filtration. We squeeze the solid parts firmly by hand so as to obtain the greatest possible amount of liquid. We then dry the remaining plant residue on a cloth or a fine net in a warm spot. We can also dry them in the sun, since the volatile constituents of the plants are gone. When the plant parts are dry, we keep them in a suitable container for later incineration and calcination, by means of which we obtain the Philosophical Salt (see page 91). We put the filtered alcoholic liquid in a fractionating flask, which is then connected with the distilling apparatus (see figure 12).

To achieve a particularly good separation of water and alcohol, we also use specific columns. Among these we find simple glass tubes that can be filled with small glass rings, as well as complicated models (see figure 19).

As the escape of the vapor is retarded in these columns, the vapor of the liquid with the higher boiling point condenses before reaching the condenser and falls back. Some columns have a vacuum jacket to

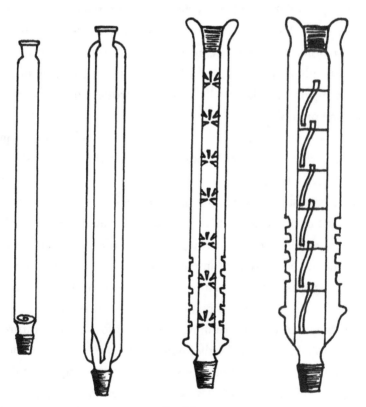

Fig. 19

guarantee a specially uniform heating. With columns without jackets, the results very much depend on the ambient temperature.

Distillation in a water or oil bath is expedient as in this way the burning of the plants, or the forming of a ring in the flask, is prevented. When distilling combustible substances, an open flame must be avoided for safety.

The boiling point of ethyl alcohol is 78° C at sea level; in higher altitudes it is somewhat lower.

At the first distilling off of our Mercury, the temperature should not exceed 85° C. When nothing more comes over, the distillation is completed.

The liquid residue in the fractionating flask is preserved. We shall later obtain the fixed Sulfur from it. (See page 85.)

An alcohol meter serves to determine the alcohol content of our distillate. It consists of a glass tube closed at both ends, one end of which is weighed by a weight, while the other has a calibrated scale. Some alcohol meters also have a built-in thermometer, since the measuring must always be done at a specific temperature (= density). The alcohol meter floats vertically in mixtures of alcohol and water. As it is calibrated to a specific temperature, the distillate must be brought to this temperature (by heating or cooling).

So we put our distillate into a sufficiently large glass measuring cylinder and carefully dip our alcohol meter into it after previously making sure of the right temperature.

The first distillate still contains a large amount of water as well as a small part of other alcohols and impurities. These are removed in the subsequent distillations. In so doing, the exact observation of and adherence to the temperature is of importance. First we discard the so-called first runnings that go over before the thermometer at the fractionating column indicates the boiling point of the ethyl alcohol, that is, 78° C. The substances of the first runnings all boil at lower temperatures than ethyl alcohol. As soon as the thermometer rises to 78° C (or shows the boiling point of ethyl alcohol corresponding to the altitude of the laboratory), we replace the receiver and remove the first runnings.

We also keep back both the remaining water and the so-called fusel oils by a precise control of the temperature. Both water and fusel oils boil at a higher temperature than ethyl alcohol, and we regulate our equipment accordingly.

The use of proper columns facilitates fractionating, that is, the separation of ethyl alcohol from the other substances. With every distillation our distillate becomes purer. After about seven distillations we get a clean ethyl alcohol of high percentage, our Mercury.

In addition, some of the impurities can be removed with a charcoal filter. Continual purifying of Mercury through repeated distillations is called rectification.

As alcohol is strongly hygroscopic, we shall hardly obtain a 100 percent concentration. Through the process of freezing we can further separate the remaining water, since water freezes at 0° but ethyl alcohol only at –114°.

In chemistry still other processes are applied. The remaining water is bound by the addition of a certain amount of calcium oxide (CaO). Then we distill again. Likewise, sodium and magnesium are used in this way. In alchemy such techniques are not permitted because they "mineralize" the alcohol. ("The tears of Diana [Mercury] are determined.")

For our purposes the way of repeated distillations, possibly with a column, such as a Vigereux column, is quite adequate. The purified Mercury (approximately 95 percent alcohol) is preserved in a tightly closed bottle.

The classical masters already had a highly developed art of distillation. They distinguished, for instance, among the following:

A. *Destillatio per ascensum* (ascending distillation), which first forced the vapors to rise before they condensed
B. *Destillatio per descensum* (descending distillation), which took the vapors immediately down without high rising
C. *Destillatio per latus* (lateral distillation), when the vapors went through a lateral horizontally affixed beak before they condensed
D. *Destillatio per inclinationem* (downward-inclined distillation), when the beak of a retort, for instance, was strongly inclined downward

Special mention is also made of the *destillatio per alembicum* (distillation over the alembic). We shall now examine various devices such as alembics.

Let us look at some classical distillation illustrations. The installation shown in figure 20 is a classical fractionating installation, consisting of a furnace with a water bath. Over the alembic with a long beak

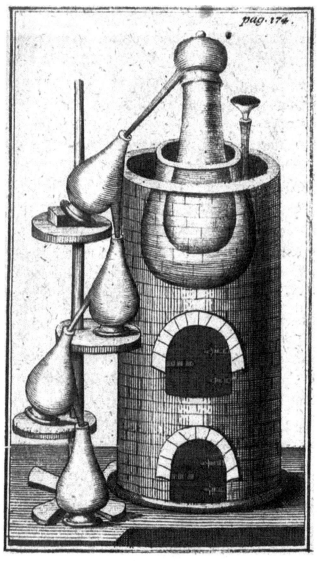

pag. 174.

Fig. 20

the vapor reaches the first (uppermost) receiver, in which part of the liquid with the highest boiling point is already condensing. The remaining vapor goes into the second, somewhat lower-lying receiver, in which part of the vapor again condenses. During the descent the temperature decreases steadily. Finally, the liquid with the lowest boiling point is collected in the bottom receiver. If we were to distill a water-alcohol mixture in this way, the water content in the uppermost receiver would be highest and the alcohol content lowest; in the bottom receiver it would be the reverse. By adaptation to the conditions of the outdoor temperature and by regulation of the distance between the receivers and the furnace, the alchemical masters achieved very precise simultaneous fractionating. The engraving in figure 20 has been taken from Johannes Isaac Hollandus's *Opera Vegetabilia* (Vienna, 1773).

Of great significance in the classical distillation are the so-called alembics. In these heads the vapors could greatly expand before their condensation. In the language of modern physics we would say the distance between the molecules was maximum.

Let us now consider some of these alembics. The engraving shown in figure 21 is taken from Andreas Libavius's work *Alchymia*, second edition (Frankfurt, 1606). We can see some *accipientia* (receptacles or recipients) and *tradentia* (transition receptacles).

The various forms of the alembic with beak, also often simply called Rostratus, are used for distilling and also for fractionating. The Coecus (blind alembic) was also used in the rotation or distillation. We shall return to it later.

Let us now consider some collecting vessels *(collectoria)* (figure 22), which we can also call recipients or receptacles. The engraving is taken from the above-quoted work of Libavius.

Now let us look at some distillation installations from Libavius's *Alchymia*. Figure 23 shows a Cinerarium or Arenarium, which is an ash-bath or sand-bath installation.

The alchemical masters distinguished between four fire grades: Grade 1 is "Mary's bath" (water bath); grade 2 is the ash bath; grade 3 is the sand bath; grade 4 is the open fire. "Distill in the second grade"

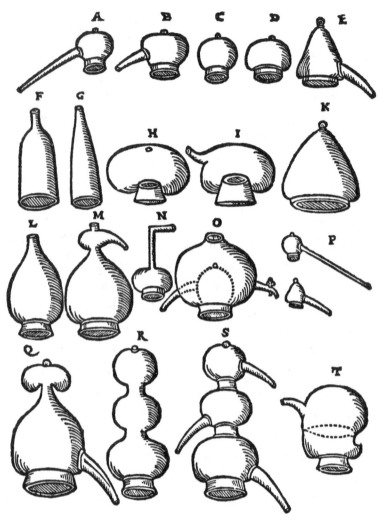

Fig. 21

(A) Alembicus rostri prolixi *(Alembic with long beak or spout)*. (B) *Alembic with short beak*. (C) *So-called blind alembic*. (D) Alembicus reductus *(reduced alembic)*. (E) Pileus *(hat)* or campana *(bell)* with beak or spout. (F) and (G) *Alembics for sublimation (dry sublimating)*. (H) Alembicus reductus *with hole*. (I) *Blind alembic with* tubulus, *which permits the addition or removal of substances*. (K) Campana *(bell)* without or with beak. (L) *"Tiara" with connecting tube*. (M) Cydaris. (N) Operculum cum syringa *(alembic with connecting tube)*. (O) Refrigerium *(alembic with water cooling)*. (P) Minuscoli *(small alembics for small distillation vessels)*. (Q) *Beak-alembic with small integrally cast blind Alembic*. (R) Coecus triplex *(triple alembic)*. (S) Rostratus triplex *(triple break alembic), a fractionating appliance*. (T) *Blind alembic similar to* (I), *with the* tubus *bent to the rear*.

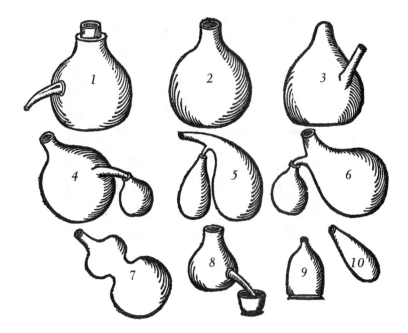

Fig. 22

(1) Flask for spirits, with beak. (2) Simple flask. (3) Excipulus coecus *(recipient with blind apex). In such flasks vapors are collected that do not easily precipitate. (4)* Excipulus geminatus *(twin recipient). (5)* Excipulus geminatus *in oblong form. (6)* Excipulus geminatus *in a somewhat different form (see figure 26). (7)* Biventer continuus *(double belly), a receiver with a greater surface for the purpose of cooling. (8) Transmission receiver. (9) and (10) Bottle-shaped receivers.*

therefore means "Distill in the ash bath." The temperatures of the ash bath are considerably higher than those of the water bath. Because of its porosity, the ash bath permits low but constant temperatures.

In figure 23, (A) is the sand bath or ash bath proper, into which the flasks are set. As ash easily flies about, it is covered, and half the flask projects. Long-beaked alembics have been put on them. The cold air took care of the cooling. (B) is the *Hypocaustum,* the combustion chamber for the fuel. (C) is the ashpit in which the ash of the fuel is collected.

The graphic representation in figure 24 is a *Distillatorium anguinum* (distillation installation with coils or spiral tubes).

It shows a water-bath distillation-installation whose first part is air-cooled, while the second part is air- and water-cooled.

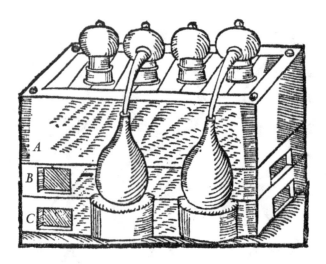

Fig. 23

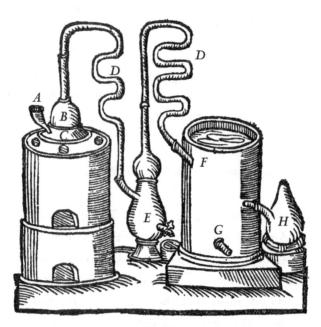

Fig. 24

(A) *Tube for the water supply.* (B) *Alembic with a connecting tube.* (C) *Neck of the water flask (also called water still).* (D) Serpentinae semicirculares *(semicircular coils).* (E) *Receptacle for the liquid with a high boiling point (watery liquid).* (F) *Entrance of the tube into the water tank.* (G) *Beak for letting out the cooling water.* (H) *Blind receptacle.*

The engraving in figure 25 shows a *stufa sicca* (dry furnace) with particularly large alembics. Such furnaces and alembics were also used for dry sublimation when no special sublimatorium was available. The much-sought-after Sal Armoniac (Salt of the Wise) could thus be collected. The furnace depicted to the right has no separate ashpit.

In figure 26 we have a so-called Pentathlum, a multipurpose appliance.

In figure 27 we have a simple fractionating installation that could be installed in a proper furnace. The appliance has a double kettle below.

Figure 28 is a so-called Abacus (actually, table): a distillation table that allows for distilling with direct heating as well as with various baths. The beaks at the lowest places of the flasks provide the watery distillates, the beaks of the alembics the subtler ones. We recognize different kinds of alembics, among them one with a branched beak. In the first receiver the watery liquid condenses, in the second the subtler.

All the installations just discussed represent fractionating equipment in one or another form. Not only were such installations used for the separation of various liquids from each other, but the decomposition

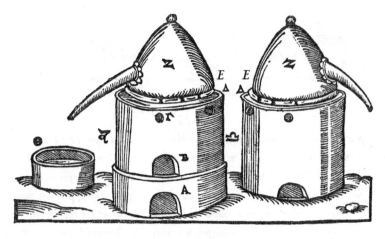

Fig. 25

(A) *Ashpit.* (B) **Hypocaustum** (*combustion chamber*). (Γ) *Airholes for regulating the heat.* (Δ) *Rim of the patina.* (E) *Rim of the alembic.* (Z) *Alembic.* (Θ) *Patella.*

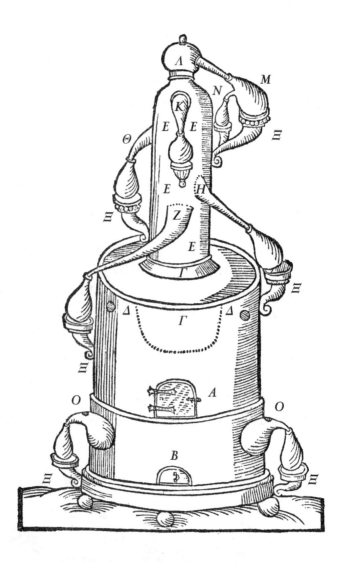

Fig. 26

(A) Hypocaustum *(combustion chamber for the fuel)*. (B) Ashpit. (Γ) Flask *(still)*
with the matter to be distilled. (Δ) *Airholes for regulating the fire*. (E) *Head with four*
beaks at various heights. (Λ) *Mounted alembic with beak for the most spiritual (i.e., the*
subtlest) waters. (Z), (H), (Θ), (K) *Beaks at various heights. The uppermost furnishes*
the subtler water, the lowest the least subtle. (M) *Collecting retort for the condensation*
of the volatile spirits, i.e., the hard-to-coagulate vapors. (N) *Receptacle for the collecting*
of the coagulated liquid. M and N together form an excipus geminus. (Ξ) *Mounting*
supports for the receivers. (O) Rectificatoria *(rectification vessels)*.

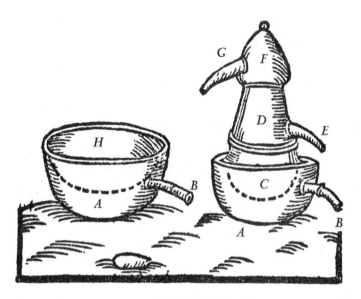

Fig. 27

(A) Lower part of the kettle for the water bath. (B) Rotatory tube for
letting water in and out. (C) Flask with beak (E). (D) Lower alembic
with (E) beak for the less subtle water. (F) Upper alembic with beak (G)
for the subtler water. (H) Inset for the reception of the flask.

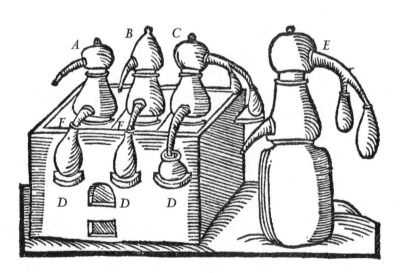

Fig. 28

of a liquid into different elements was thereby also realized. Now a few words concerning this matter.

According to the alchemists, there exist different kinds of distilled water. During distillation the total quantity of the water to be distilled is divided into four Elements. That is, distill 1,000 milliliters of water into four 250-ml batches. The first 25 percent of the total quantity that flows into the receiver are designated as the "fire of the water." This amount (250 ml) represents the subtlest part of the water. In the case of a simultaneous distillation with the above-described Pentathlum we would look for the fire of the water at the upper beak (K). The second 25 percent form the "air of the water," the third 25 percent are the "water of the water," and the last 25 percent form the "earth of the water," which we would look for at the lowest beak when using the Pentathlum. An appliance like the Pentathlum permits simultaneous fractionating. But we can also decompose a quantity of water by a successive separation of the Elements. To do this, slow distillation ("sweating over") is required, which allows the individual Elements to come forth one after another. The decomposition of the water takes place automatically with right heating, provided the exact quantities are adhered to.

Decomposition can be continued further.

Each of the distilled Elements can now be decomposed into the three Essentials, that is, into the three Philosophical Principles.

If we distill our 250 ml of "fire of the water," we first obtain one-third (83.33 ml) of Mercury, then one-third of Sulfur, and finally one-third of Salt.

If we also continue the decomposition with the other Elements, we finally obtain four different Mercuries (one from each Element), four different Sulfurs, and four different Salia or Salts.

The Coagula (the joining of the separated constituents) of this work is now done in such a way that first all Mercuries are poured together, then all Sulfurs, and finally all Salia. Finally the three Essentials are again poured together, that is, first Mercury into Sal, then Sulfur into this mixture.

The accompanying diagram shows the process once again. As original material, thunderstorm water is recommended, for it "carries within itself the heavenly fire." That is, rainwater collected during a thunderstorm with lightning. First, ☿ is poured into ⊖, then the ♃. (The ⊖ is enlivened and animated, or supplied with a soul.)

A. 1 L	B.1	B.2	B.3	B.4	C.
Thunderstorm water fractionated into:	250 ml △	250 ml ⩟	250 ml ▽	250 ml ⩞	Poured together
	This in 83.33 ml ☿	This in 83.33 ml ☿	This in 83.33 ml ☿	This in 83.33 ml ☿	= 333.33 ml ☿
	83.33 ml ♃	83.33 ml ♃	83.33 ml ♃	83.33 ml ♃	= 333.33 ml ♃
	83.33 ml ⊖	83.33 ml ⊖	83.33 ml ⊖	83.33 ml ⊖	= 333.33 ml ⊖

During the entire process we work exclusively with water. The above-described work is the production of a so-called Archaeus[37] out of water, which is then used for specific purposes. The quality of the fractions of the water differs somewhat from one to another. This can be proved by a sensitive analysis.

Modern science smiles at such experiments. Water alchemy, however, is a specialized field to which many of the alchemical masters devoted a great deal of time. Knowledge of the qualities of different waters is indispensable for many magisteries. For some May dew is prescribed, for others thunderstorm water. Lightning indeed transforms part of the nitrogen in the air into nitrogen compounds, which then reach the earth together with the rain. In this way every field receives a certain amount of fertilizer free of charge.

The last engraving from Libavius shows the use of solar energy (figure 29). To the left we see a closed flask that is exposed to the rays of the sun reflected by a concave mirror. It is a matter of a circulation or digestion caused by the reflection of the sunbeams.

To the right we see a similar container that is exposed to the rays of the sun focused through a lens. Here an exaltation by refraction takes place. In the center we see a distillation by reflection of the sunbeams. If

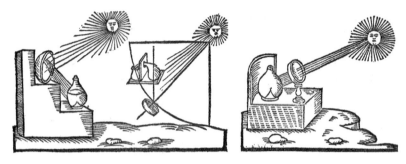

Fig. 29

we bear in mind that the alchemical masters did not even have the use of a thermometer, we must admire their distilling art, because they achieved quite difficult magisteries with relatively simple equipment. By experience the ancients had developed a very precise sensitiveness. Intuition and precise observation replaced the measuring instruments. At that same time Stradivari and Guarneri built their masterly musical instruments with very simple technical devices but with the greatest expertise. Their instruments have remained unequaled even to this day.

Did the masters know vacuum distillation?

Basilius Valentinus writes in his *Triumphal Chariot of Antimony:* "and from the bath of the holy chaste Virgin Mary distill the vinegar down until a red-yellow, dry powder remains."[38] And in another passage: "But this I tell you, when such an extraction is drawn out with the vinegar, and the vinegar is distilled off in the Women's Bath, and thereafter the remaining powder is resolved in loco humido. . . ."[39]

Could vinegar, whose boiling point is 118° C, be distilled in the water bath at 100° C? It is only possible in a vacuum. (In regard to using a vacuum, one must be careful not to draw out, through the pump, the essence sought for!)

Perhaps we now understand the significance of the fish bladder in the hand of the old man in figure 6. We have no further proof, and it would serve no useful purpose to indulge in speculation. Let us rather return to the continuation of our work.

Fixed Sulfur and Its Salt

To obtain fixed Sulfur, we must evaporate the plant soup that remains after the distillation of Mercury. In this way we obtain a viscous mass reminiscent of honey or pitch, depending on the degree of the evaporation. We shall call it honey in the following comments. This honey is the fixed vegetable honey.

It is only seldom used in this form; much more frequent is the use of the salts of the Sulfur, simply called "salts of Sulfur."

The salts of Sulfur, of which some are water-soluble, others insoluble in water, are obtained through incineration and subsequent calcination of the honey. Consequently, we put our honey into a suitable evaporating container such as a flameproof or heat-resistant glass dish and slowly heat it on a gas flame or electric hotplate.

A process interesting to observe now begins: the honey gradually turns darker and starts to throw bubbles and sputter. The contents of the dish look like a volcanic mass. A strong formation of smoke with a pungent smell evolves, and yellowish vapors escape from the bubbles bursting on the surface. The mass becomes ever more subdued, until finally everything is black and hard. The whole spectacle strongly reminds us of volcanic activity, and after observing this we can understand why the mass is called Sulfur. We now increase the temperature of the heating, and gradually our vegetable Sulfur carbonizes. When it becomes quite hard, we can also grind it in a mortar. The carbonized fixed Sulfur is then calcined.

In the language of chemistry, calcination means the decomposition of a chemico-organic compound through heat, while driving off carbon dioxide and water. In the language of alchemy, calcination means "making white like chalk." The Greek word for calcination is *titanosis* from *titanos*, "chalk."

Right calcination requires much sensitiveness and experience. A number of mistakes can be made. If the temperature is too low, the calcination does not make headway; with too-high temperatures, certain components of the material being calcined will fuse. At the bottom of the flameproof dish we can then recognize a metallic-looking dark spot. A long calcination at relatively low temperatures (400°–500° C) is always preferable to a brief violent one. At approximately 900° C the water-soluble salts melt, which would spoil the whole work. Frequently, calcining takes place continuously for several days.

Thus the black mass gradually changes into a grayish-white ash. Alchemically viewed, calcination is a purification and pulverization by means of fire.

Should it happen that our calcination temperature inadvertently gets too high and part of the salts melt, we can nevertheless save the situation by a clever method. Let us listen to some pertinent words by Johannes Isaac Hollandus:[40]

> But should it happen that you heated too much through carelessness and the earth [in this text, the designation for the calcining matter] began to melt and turned into glass, your work would nevertheless not be totally spoiled, but you would have to take it out, grind it small in an iron mortar, and subsequently grind it impalpably (quite fine) on stone with distilled vinegar, put it in a stone pot, pour on it distilled vinegar, and set it in the Balneum [water bath] for one day and night, then take it out, let it sink [let the solid parts settle], filter, and again pour vinegar upon the Feces [the residue on the filter], stir, and again put it for one day in the Balneum, then remove and filter it, and put everything together into a pot, and again set it in the Balneum, and draw off the vinegar [distill in the water bath under vacuum] until your earth is dry; then you have your earth back out of the Fecibus, now dissolve it again once or twice in your water [distilled water], should there be more Feces in it.

The feces are here the salts that are insoluble in water that are eliminated simultaneously with the correction of the wrong calcination. We shall return later to the meaning of the word *earth* in this context. As is evident, the correction just mentioned is not so simple. It therefore pays to observe the right temperature.

The alchemical masters distinguished between open and closed calcination (*calcinatio aperta* and *calcinatio occlusa*). With open calcination some of the volatile components are lost, among them, for instance, Sal Armoniacum, which is indispensable for some magisteries.[41] With closed calcination the whole process goes on hermetically sealed.

The ancients performed the closed calcination within a thick clay ball, which had to be firm and leakproof on all sides. There were also specific furnaces in which a heated chamber could be tightly sealed off. In these chambers the substances were calcined without a clay cover. When the clay ball was used, it was put into the open fire. It was to be surrounded on all sides by heat. (This procedure is widely used in Judaic alchemical work.) Especially convenient for this work were the so-called reverberating furnaces, in which the flames could also sweep over the substances from above. The heating up had to be done gradually, and both the clay ball and its content had to be as dry as possible. We shall now consider three classical calcining furnaces. The illustrations are taken from the previously mentioned *Alchymia* by Andreas Libavius.

Figure 30 shows us two simple calcining furnaces. Model B has a separate ash compartment under the heating chamber. Figure 31 pictures a round calcining furnace. Figure 32 shows a covered calcining furnace.

In an electric enameling stove, closed calcination can easily be carried out by enclosing the calcining material between two identical, approximately hemispherical clay crucibles. The flat edges are cemented together with clay or loam or else secured with a strong clamp or wire.

For the open calcination we spread the carbonized substance evenly over the bottom of the flameproof dish and heat from below. Slowly the contents of the container become grayish-white. Calcination often lasts several days; a slow oxidation process takes place. We leave the container safely on the stove and slowly observe the discoloration. When the white color does not get brighter, even after prolonged heating, the calcination is done. We turn the heating off and let the matter cool down. We now have before us the salts of the Sulfur.

Often we can speed up the whitening by a clever technique: we sprinkle the gray ash with distilled water, then we calcine again.

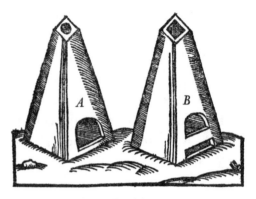

Fig. 30

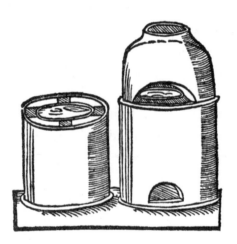

Fig. 31

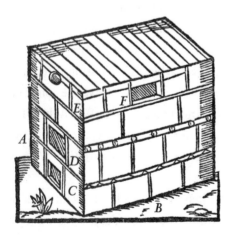

Fig. 32
A covered calcining furnace.
(A) Front view. (B) Side view.
(C) Ash pit. (D) Heating chamber.
(E) Calcining space. (F) Access.

The two salts of Sulfur, the water-soluble one and that which is insoluble in water, must be separated from each other. To do this, we pour approximately triple the quantity of distilled water over the white ash and stir well. If necessary, we heat slightly, or we let everything stand in moderate heat for a whole night. Subsequently, we filter the solution. The filtrate is transparent and almost colorless. To obtain all water-soluble salts, we must wash the feces several times with fresh distilled water, filtering each time. The filtrate is always added to the previously extracted salt solution.

We can obtain a practically total extraction with the Soxhlet process discussed further below.

Finally, the salts that are insoluble in water remain. They are also called Caput Mortuum (Death's Head) and are not further used in many magisteries.

The filtrate containing the water-soluble salts is corrosive on the tongue. It is strongly alkaline, and litmus paper is immediately colored intensely blue when moistened with it.

To make the water-soluble salts visible, we now evaporate the salt solution slowly at low temperatures, for example, in the sun or on a radiator. (Protect it from dust.) When all the water has evaporated, we find a white salt at the bottom of the container. It is the water-soluble salt of the Sulfur, also called the salt proper of the Sulfur. The salt is strongly hygroscopic. In the open, humid air it would liquefy in a short time, and we therefore put it in a tightly closed glass for storage.

It happens occasionally that the salt solution extracted from the calcined ash shows a yellowish-orange streak that can go as far as a brownish tint. In this case the duration of the calcination was not adequate, and we must calcine the salt once more after drying it. Then we dissolve it again in distilled water, filter, and then let the water evaporate anew. We may have to repeat this process several times. Finally, we have a pure white salt.

If we wish also to purify the salts that are insoluble in water, we must wash them in distilled water until the litmus paper no longer shows any alkaline reaction; that is, the litmus paper must not indicate a higher pH-value than that of the water used for rinsing. The salt that is insoluble in water is now also dried; sputtering need not be feared, and that is why our temperature can be higher. The melting point, too, is so high (about 1600° C) that there is no danger of unintentional melting. At the end we have before us a light gray powder that is not hygroscopic and has a limelike taste. We put it into a suitable glass for storage.

To separate the water-soluble salts from those that are insoluble we can also use a Soxhlet Extractor (figure 33).

The white calcined ash is put into a paper thimble, which is then set into the extraction chamber (A) of the Soxhlet Extractor.

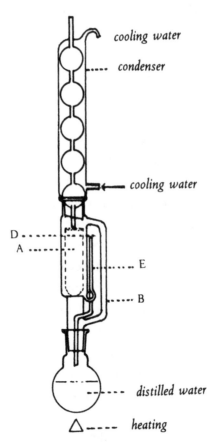

Fig. 33

In the glass flask below there is distilled water. Upon the extractor is mounted a condenser (it usually comes with the appliance), through which the cooling water flows. Now we heat the flask. When the temperature of the water reaches the boiling point, the vapor rises into the condenser through tube B, where it condenses at once and drips into the filled extraction thimble in the form of water. Slowly the surface of the liquid rises in the extraction chamber A; as soon as it reaches point D, a reflux of the salt solution follows automatically into the flask over the siphon D, and the whole process begins anew. As only the water evaporates, the content of the extraction thimble is continually washed, causing the solution in the flask to become more concentrated with every overflow. If the temperature and the flow of the cooling water have once been regulated, we can leave the equipment to work unattended for a longer period. Finally, we evaporate the concentrated solution in the flask, as mentioned before, and in this way obtain our water-soluble salts of Sulfur. Those that are insoluble in water remain in the extraction thimble. We remove the thimble from the extractor and dry the contents to a light gray powder, which we keep as the Caput Mortuum of the Sulfur.

Salt

We obtain the Salt proper, also called Sal Salis (Salt of the Salt), representing the third Philosophical Principle, from the remaining solid plant residue. For this reason it is also called the Salt of the Body, while the Sal Sulphuris (Salt of Sulfur) is also designated as Salt of the Soul.

Our now-dry plant residues are therefore first reduced to ash in a flameproof dish, and the ash is subsequently calcined. After this, the water-soluble salts are separated from those that are insoluble in water through extraction with distilled water. (The solution is filtered, and the water-soluble salts are prepared by careful evaporation of the water.) The process is the same as that described in connection with the preparation of the salts of Sulfur: again we obtain a white, strongly hygroscopic salt (the Salt proper), and a certain amount of light gray Caput Mortuum. We preserve both substances in closed glasses.

Our separation of the plant into its three Philosophical Principles is completed.

There they now stand in front of us, the three Essentials of our plant, in their purified form. We store them in six different glasses.

What have we obtained?

1. *Mercury,* a pure, high-proof plant spirit, an alcohol that is volatile and colorless.

Mercury connects and mediates. Water as well as essential oils are soluble in ethyl alcohol, while the essential oils float on top of the water. As Mercury generates both, they all dissolve into one another, just as metals (iron excepted) dissolve into quicksilver. With quicksilver we can amalgamate metals. Ethyl alcohol "amalgamates" in the plant world and is therefore considered the Mercury or the quicksilver of the plant kingdom.

2. *Sulfur,* which consists of a volatile and a fixed (solid) part.

Essential oil forms the volatile part of Sulfur. This oil has an immediately recognizable intensive smell, characteristic of the plant from which it stems. The essential oil is, so to speak, the essence of the "personality" of the plant concerned. The volatile essential oil is combustible. It is heat-related, which can be recognized by the diathermy discussed on page 56.

From the fixed Sulfur we have prepared the salts of Sulfur: a white, water-soluble salt that is strongly hygroscopic and corrosive on the tongue, and a salt that is insoluble in water and light gray, the Caput Mortuum of the fixed Sulfur, which is not hygroscopic and has a lime-like taste.

We could also have preserved the fixed Sulfur in the form of evaporated "honey." But this is only used in a few preparations. In some magisteries it is important for the volatilization of the Sal Salis. We shall return to it in the discussion of the Circulatum Minus.

3. *The bipartite Salt.* As with the Salt of Sulfur, we have gotten a water-soluble one, the Sal Salis, and one that is insoluble in water, the Caput Mortuum of the Salt. The water-soluble one is white like that of the Sulfur, is hygroscopic, and tastes corrosive; the Caput Mortuum of

the Salt is light gray and tastes limelike, just like that of the Sulfur.

If we have worked correctly, we can obtain an idea of the quantities of the Philosophical Principles we can expect of a plant by weighing the substances accurately. We record these quantities in writing, so as to compare them with the data from other plants. Of course, we can only determine the quantity of Mercury to be expected if we have fermented with sugar.

The exact keeping of a laboratory diary should be the duty of every practicing spagyrist.

We have now effected the Solve. What about the Coagula? We shall hear about it in chapter 11. In the meantime, we will carefully preserve our Philosophical Principles.

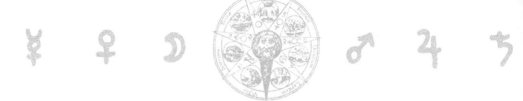

6
THE STARS

The stars are healed by the stars.

—Paracelsus

The Foundations

Paracelsus was of the opinion that every physician should simultaneously be an alchemist and an astrologer:

> Therefore he must judge the medicine according to the stars, in order to understand the higher and the lower stars. Medicine is without value if it is not from Heaven; it must be from Heaven. . . .
>
> For example, everything concerning the brain is brought to the brain by the moon, everything concerning the heart is brought to it by the sun. In this manner the kidneys are ruled by Venus, the liver by Jupiter, the gall by Mars. [*Paragranum*]

What does Paracelsus consider to be astrology?

> Astrology. This science teaches and interprets according to the whole of the firmament, how its relations are to the earth and man, according to the original order, and what is the relation between man, the earth, and the stars. [*Hermetic Astronomy*]

Astrology is closely linked with alchemy. Both sciences work with common symbols. Thus, for instance, planetary signs are used for metals in alchemistic texts: ☉ for gold, ☽ for silver, ☿ for quicksilver, ♀ for copper, ♁ for antimony, ♂ for iron, ♃ for tin, and ♄ for lead.

Both sciences see the effect of archetypal forces behind the spirit-soul-material manifestation of the universe, which form the foundation of the order (the "original order" of Paracelsus). The Solve of alchemy, which decomposes the *Mixti* (all things in the universe that are composed of more than one substance) into single constituents, presents many parallels with analytical astrology. On the other hand, the Coagula of alchemy is ever the great synthesis, which fits the separate constituents back into the whole, just as in the last analysis astrology represents a holistic view that considers both the separate organs and forces in man in their reciprocal action and the whole of man in connection with the cosmos.

Nobody can seriously doubt that there exists a connection between all single things in the universe. Astrology is studying these connections to make them available to cognition and prediction. In this respect astrology has much in common with meteorology.

Here now are some examples.

A special sensation was created by the studies about the "moon punctuality" of the palolo worm that dwells in the coral reefs of the Samoa, Fiji, Tonga, and Gilbert islands. The inhabitants of these islands equip their boats twice a year to experience a spectacle that is repeated with astronomical punctuality.

In the early-morning hours before daybreak, on the day before the last quarter of the moon in October and November, the approximately 25-centimeter-long abdomens of the worms' bodies become detached and swarm to the surface of the sea, where the evacuation and assimilation of germinal matters take place. The enormous hordes of mollusks, considered delicacies, need only be scooped up by the fishermen.

J. Goldborough Mayer has observed that *Eunice furcata*, another type of mollusk in the Atlantic Ocean near Florida, reaches sexual maturity in July, when the crisis occurs at the first or last quarter of the moon.

At the time of the full moon, the ovaries of the sea urchins of the

Mediterranean reach their maximum growth. During 1920–1921, Henry Monroe Fox devoted himself in Suez to the investigation of the lunar periodicity in the reproduction of *Centrechinus setosus*.[42] Significant are also the experiments that L. Kolisko has carried out in connection with seed germination as also with the capillar-dynamolitic examination of specific metallic salts and planetary positions.[43] The charts obtained by this method show marked changes at the time of the conjunctions of the planet that rules the corresponding salts when compared with the charts that did not arise during the conjunctions. The results of these examinations are of double importance: not only could the relation between planets and metallic salts be proved, but the results are at the same time evidence that the connection of metals with specific planets, as it was taught by the ancients, is right; because the change in the charts during the conjunctions clarifies the connection between lead and Saturn, between silver and the Moon, tin and Jupiter, and gold and the Sun.

About twenty-seven years ago, the French statistician Michel Gauquelin began his collection of ten thousand astrological data from medical doctors, politicians, sportsmen, artists, and members of the armed forces, with the aim of refuting astrological ideas. In spite of his publicly admitted negative attitude toward astrology, this investigation ended with a confession of positive, statistically provable findings that support astrology.[44] Gauquelin's investigations likewise support the view held by astrology that hereditary factors can be recognized in a horoscope. He has discovered statistically important connections between the astrological positions of parents and children.

Too high a valuation of statistics alone may be problematic in connection with the stratification and the infinite possibilities of variation of the planetary positions. It would be presumptuous to believe that such a differentiated consideration as the astrological rests only on statistics, since every horoscope belongs to an individual personality. Nevertheless, statistical investigations in this connection have their worth, at least in part.

Dr. Eugen Jonas, director of the Institute for Birth Control, supported by the Czechoslovak government, has proved that a method of astrological birth control is 97.7 percent reliable. Based on the position of the moon at the time of conception, he has also developed a method for predicting the sex of an unborn child.

John H. Nelson, electro-engineer at RCA, has discovered that magnetic storms harmful to health occur when planets stand at angles of 0°, 90°, and 180° to each other. In connection with measurements of radio interference, he has proved that interference-free fields are produced when planets form angles of 60° and 120°.

Professor Helmut Berg at the University of Cologne has discovered that times of magnetic disturbances and solar eruptions are periods when pulmonary diseases and hemorrhages are critical.

Professor H. Bertels of Berlin has discovered that microbiotic reactions, changes in the weather, and chemical reactions are connected with solar flares.

Professor A. L. Tchijensky at the University of Moscow and later Dr. Robert O. Becker of the Syracuse Veterans Hospital have discovered that historic epidemics of typhus, cholera, smallpox, and the plague occurred at the time of maximum sunspot activity.

Dr. Maki Takata of Toho University, Tokyo, could prove that the composition of human blood changes with the eleven-year sunspot rhythm. A change also occurs during the daily rotation of the earth, for which sunrise is especially important. "Man is a living sundial."

Dr. Abraham Hoffer of the University Clinic in Saskatchewan, Canada, has discovered that neurotics have particularly intense experiences in January and July; depressives in March.

In 1970, Jan Gerhard Toonder and John Anthony West began the attempt to critically examine astrology. Here now is their verdict after the conclusion of their research. They say, "It is becoming increasingly difficult to avoid the impression that Pythagoras, Plato, Plotinus, Ptolemy, Thomas Aquinas, Albertus Magnus, and Johannes Kepler were right in their assessment of astrology, at least in principle, while all of modern science is wrong."[45]

The situation of astrology is not unlike that of serious alchemy. Many old views are now confirmed by modern research, whereby old symbolic concepts are often replaced by modern ideas and discussed in a language adapted to those ideas. Whether this always brings about a clarification is another question.

After all that has been said, it seems natural that spagyrics leans closely on cosmic rhythms.

Astrology is consulted:

1. For the diagnosis of the diseases to be treated. Medical astrology is too wide a field to be dealt with here. The reader is advised to refer to the works cited in the bibliography.
2. For the classification of medicinal plants. Every medicinal plant possesses the powers of specific planets to a more or less greater degree. As with certain organs in the human body, certain parts of plants can come under the influence of one specific planet, others under that of another planet, although one or two planets always rule the whole plant. A species is therefore always classified according to the strongest influence. In this connection alchemists speak of the Doctrine of Signatures.[46]
3. In the preparation of tinctures, essences, circulata, and so on, especially at the beginning of the work, the spagyrist conforms to the planetary rhythms. Specific signs of the zodiac and their ruling planets are connected with specific works. In some cases, the positions of the moon are of significance (particularly in plant spagyrics); in others, the so-called planetary hours are important; for others again, the precise horoscope of the moment is consulted.
4. For the determination of the most favorable time for the administration of the remedy.

Even if spagyric preparations are therapeutic per se, "going with the stars" can improve the results, according to the traditional view. It is the same with sailing. Even with little wind one can make headway by clever maneuvers, but things go better with a more favorable wind and the proper sail.

For all that, we should always listen to the view that says that the "plane above the stars" can be reached through absolute seriousness and devotion. Paracelsus says that the highest form of medicine is love. In this case medicine can become free of *karma*. In this connection, we shall cite yet another sentence often quoted among astrologers: "The wise rule the stars."

Let us now turn to the seven planets of the ancients, the signs of the zodiac, and the corresponding order of the medicinal plants.

Beyond Saturn, the "Guardian of the Threshold," the "octaves" begin, to which belong Uranus, Neptune, Pluto, and not yet officially discovered planets.

The ancients divided the planets into "benefactors" and "malefactors." They likewise spoke of "good" or "evil" aspects. Modern astrology prefers the designations "synthetic" and "analytic" aspects.

Before we turn to the rhythms, let us survey the planets and their zodiacal signs with the organs, plants, and works belonging to them.

Stars and Medicinal Plants

☉ *The Sun*

As the center of our solar system, the Sun contains the elements from which plants were formed in a highly ionized form (plasma stage), that is, in the fourth state of aggregation of matter.

All life is sustained by the radiation of light and warmth from the Sun.

The Sun generates extraordinarily strong magnetic fields. According to the findings of the *Pioneer* (deep space probe) expeditions, the Sun's magnetic field reaches the orbit of Pluto in the form of a solar wind.

Depending on their size and elements, the individual planets transform solar energy into specific energy flows that then reach the earth.

For example, solar energy is partly manifested by electricity, which is solar power reflected by the planet Uranus.

The Sun rules the mind and willpower, energy, vitality, wholeness and self-integration, dominion, organization, and power in general.

Physiologically, the Sun rules the heart, circulation, the vertebral column, health and vitality in general, and the heart meridian of acupuncture; in addition, the distribution of heat in the body, the thymus gland, the *pons Varolii* (function: control of the breath), and the eyes (especially the right eye of man and the left of woman). Together with Saturn and the signs of Virgo and Scorpio, the Sun rules the spleen. The energies transformed by the spleen are carried to the solar plexus, from where they spread over the whole body. (Compare the significance and function of the spleen for energy economy in Chinese medicine.)

The image of the Sun is masculine, conscious, and libido-like.

The diseases associated with the Sun are organic, constitutional, and structural.

The Sun's metal is gold (in the Indian view also copper). Its zodiacal sign is the Lion.

Its fragrance is olibanum incense, its precious stones are the cat's eye *(chrysolith)* and, in the Indian view, the ruby.

Plants That Come Especially under the Dominion of the Sun

Althaea officinalis: marshmallow (with Jupiter and Venus)

Anagallis arvensis: common scarlet pimpernel (with Jupiter)

Angelica archangelica: angelica, lingwort (with Venus)

Angelica silvestris: wild angelica (with Venus)

Anthemis nobilis: Roman chamomile

Calamus aromaticus (Acorus calamus): calamus

Calendula officinalis: marigold

Caryophyllus (Syzygium aromaticum): clove tree

Chelidonium majus: celandine (with Jupiter)

Cinnamonum ceylanicum: cinnamon, Ceylon cinnamon

Citrus aurantium: orange tree

Citrus bergamium: bergamot

Citrus limonum: lemon tree

Dictamnus albus: dittany

Drosera rotundifolia: sundew

Echium valgare: viper's buglass, blueweed

Erythrea centaurium (Entaurium umbellatum): lesser centaury

Euphrasia officinalis: eyebright
Fragaria vesca: wild strawberry (with Jupiter)
Fraxinus excelsior: ash (with Jupiter)
Gentiana lutea: gentian (with Jupiter)
Glechoma hederacea: ground ivy (with Venus)
Helianthus anuus: sunflower
Hypericum perforatum: Saint-John's-wort
Inula helenium: elecampane
Juglans regia: walnut tree (with Mercury)
Juniperus communis: juniper (with Jupiter and Mercury)
Laurus nobilis: laurel (with Jupiter)
Matricaria chamomilla: German chamomile
Melissa officinalis: lemon balm (with Jupiter)
Olea europea: olive tree (with Jupiter; often classified under Jupiter)
Oryza sativa: rice
Paeonia officinalis: peony
Passiflora incarnata: passionflower
Piper: pepper (white and black)
Plantago lanceolata: ribwort (with Mars)
Plantago major: plantain (with Mars)
Potentilla reptans: cinquefoil, five-leaf, finger-grass
Rosmarinus officinalis: rosemary
Ruta graveolens: common rue
Sinapis alba: white mustard
Sinapis nigra: black mustard
Viscum album: mistletoe (with Jupiter and moon)
Vitis vinifera: grapevine (with Jupiter and moon)
Zedoaria (Curcuma zedoaria): zedoary
Zingiber officinale: ginger

The entire family of the labiates is heat- and Sun-related; likewise, and especially, the essential oils that represent volatile Sulfur (Apollo).

Therapeutic effects of the solar plants are toning up, heating, and diaphoretic, affecting the circulation, heart, thymus, spleen, and eyes.

☽ *The Moon*

The Moon is the only satellite of the Earth. It reflects the light and other energies of the Sun, which it gathers and carries through the twelve signs of the zodiac during a synodical month.

The Moon influences the water on the Earth through high and low tides. The new moon and the full moon cause high tide, while the flood stays lower during the quarters of the moon.

At the Full Moon the chances for hemorrhages and births increase. At the New Moon nocturnal activity is slight; at the Full Moon it is great.

The Moon influences growth, fertility, conception, the subconscious, the feelings, rhythms, instincts, reflection, passivity, motherliness, family, and heritage.

Subject to the Moon are the stomach and the esophagus, the breasts, the womb and the ovaries, menstruation, the body fluids (e.g., the blood serum), the urinary bladder, the cerebellum, the pancreas, and the memory.

The Moon is related to the eyes (to the left eye of man and the right eye of woman), the brain, saliva, glandular secretion, sensuality, the thyroid gland (with Mercury and the sign of Scorpio), the tonsils (with the sign of Taurus), the lachrymal mechanism, and the transformation of fluids.

The Moon's image is feminine, changeable, motherly, familiar. Bright and dark traits are mixed, on the one hand benevolence and motherliness, on the other wildness and raw instincts. The Moon has a dark side.

Diseases associated with the Moon are periodically recurring illnesses, irregular menses, as well as diseases of the lunar organs. At the Full Moon epileptics, somnambulists, and hysterical or nervous persons are influenced unfavorably.

Lunar metals and minerals are silver, moonstone (selenite), pearls, and amber.

Scents are melon, jasmine (according to another view, jasmine has more Jovian qualities), hyssop, and poppy. The zodiacal sign is Cancer.

Plants That Come Especially under the Dominion of the Moon

The whole plant world is especially subject to the moon.

> *Penetrating into the earth, I sustain all creatures by My strength; By becoming the moon full of juices, I nourish all plants.*
>
> [BHAGAVAD GĪTĀ, 15:13]

Especially strongly lunar are:

Acanthus mollis: acanthus
Agnus castus: monk's pepper
Atriplex silvestris: atriplex, orache, all-seed, notchweed
Bellis perennis: daisy
Brassicae: all kinds of cabbage, brassicaceous plants
Cardamine pratense: lady's smock, cuckoo flower
Carica papaya: papaya
Cheiranthus cheiri: wallflower
Cucumis sativus: cucumber
Cucurbita Pepo: pumpkin, gourd
Curcuma longa: turmeric
Galium aparine: galium, cleavers, goose grass
Hieracium pilosella: hawkweed, mouse-ear
Hyssopus officinalis: hyssop
Iris florentina: Florentine iris (with Saturn)
Iris germanica: German iris (with Saturn), dark blue flowers
Iris pallida: pale iris (with Saturn), pale blue flowers
Lactuca sativa: cabbage-lettuce
Lenticula palustris: duckweed
Ligustrum vulgare: privet
Lilium album: white lily
Lysimachia nummularia: moneywort
Myristica fragrans: nutmeg

Nasturtium officinale: watercress
Nymphaea alba: water lily
Papaver rhoeas: corn poppy (with Saturn)
Papaver somniferum: opium poppy (with Saturn)
Ruta lunaria: moonwort
Salices: all kinds of willows
Saxifraga: saxifrage
Sedum acre: sharp stonecrop, wall-pepper
Sedum telephium: orpine
Stellaria media: chickweed
Telephium vulgare: sedum
Tilia: lime-tree (with Venus)
Trapa natans: water chestnut
Veronica officinalis: speedwell
Vinca minor: myrtle, periwinkle

Therapeutic effect of the lunar plants: many food plants, alterative, cooling, moisturizing, enzymic, and promoting fermentation.

☿ *Mercury*

Of all the planets, Mercury is nearest to the Sun. In horoscopes it can never be farther than 28° from the Sun, and it is therefore only visible as the morning or evening star. The magnetic field of Mercury resembles that of the Earth. The planet reflects the light of the Sun, infrared rays, and radio waves, like the Moon.

Its period of revolution is 59.65 days = two synodic months, its time of rotation around the Sun = three synodic months.

Mercury is the mediator, the messenger of the gods; the Romans also considered Mercury the god of commerce.

As a hermaphrodite he stands between the polarized sexes, ambivalent and unreliable, dry and cold if masculine, humid and cold if feminine.

As the Egyptian Hermes Trismegistus (Thoth), he invented language and writing and ranked as the patron of the medical art.

Under Mercury come the intellect, mediation, transmission, and translation, mental and nervous processes, speech and writing, dexterity, ambivalence, and the distribution of energies.

The planet rules the nervous system (with Uranus), the ears, hearing, the tongue, speech, the vocal organs; especially the nerves of the arms, the abdomen, the cerebrospinal nerves of the brain (with the Moon), the bronchia, respiration, coordination between body and mind, reason, the feet, the nerves of the sex and urinary organs, the thyroid, the hands, the legs, and the heart, the optical nerve, the invisible "nerve fluids," the motor nerves, the larynx, the lungs, the mental abilities (with the Moon, Uranus, and Neptune), and the spinal cord. The Sun-like cerebrum and the Moon-like cerebellum are linked by the Mercurial pons.

Mercury has its image as the messenger of the gods, the healer, and mediator, but also as the planetary genius of magic and trickery. Its symbols are the winged sandals and the caduceus.

The diseases associated with Mercury are mainly disturbances that are in each case connected with the organs ruled by the zodiacal signs in which the planet is at the time. As the planet is capable of changing, the kind of disturbance greatly depends on the other planets with which Mercury is connected.

Metals and minerals of Mercury are quicksilver, topaz, opal, tourmaline, peridot, and, in the view of the Indians and also of Agrippa, the emerald.

Mercurial scents are all kinds of wormwood, narcissus, anise, and parsley. Its zodiacal signs are Gemini and Virgo.

Plants That Come Especially under the Dominion of Mercury

Adiantum capillus veneris: maidenhair
Acacia: all kinds of acacias
Alliaria officinalis: garlic, hedge-mustard
Anethum graveolens: dill
Apium graveolens: celery
Artemisia abrotanum: southernwood
Artemisia absinthium: wormwood (with Venus)

Avena sativa: oats (with Jupiter)

Azalea: azalea

Bryonia alba: bryony

Calamintha montana: calamint, mountain balm, wild basil

Calamintha arvensis: mint, calamint

Carum carvi: caraway

Chichorium endivia: endive, chicory

Convallaria majalis: lily-of-the-valley (with the Moon)

Corylus avella: hazel

Cynoglossum officinale: hound's tongue (with Jupiter)

Daucus carota: carrot

Digitalis purpurea: digitalis, red foxglove

Foeniculum vulgare: fennel

Glycyrrhiza glabra: licorice

Inula helenium: elecampane

Lavandula vera: lavender (with Jupiter and the Sun)

Lonicera caprifolium: honeysuckle, woodbine

Majorana hortensis: marjoram (with the Sun)

Mandragora: mandrake (with Saturn and the Moon)

Marrubium vulgare: horehound, white

Mercurialis annua: mercury, annual

Mercurialis perennis: perennial mercury

Morus alba: mulberry tree, white

Morus nigra: mulberry tree, black

Myrtus communis: myrtle

Origanum vulgare: oregano, origanum

Parietaria officinalis: wall pellitory

Pastinaca sativa: parsnip

Petroselinum hortense: parsley

Pimpinella anisum: anise

Piper cubeba: cubeb pepper

Satureja hortensis: savory

Solanum dulcamara: bittersweet

Strychnos flux vomica: vomic or poison nut

Teucrium scordium: germander
Trifolium arvense: harefoot, hop trefoil, hopclover
Trifolium fibrinum: marsh trefoil, buckbean
Tussilago farfara: coltsfoot
Valeriana officinalis: valerian

Typical effects of Mercurial medicinal plants are changes of mind, effects on the brain and the nervous system, and menstruation-regulating effects.

♀ *Venus*

Venus is approximately as big as the Earth. Its longest distance from the sun is 47°. Through its dense carbon dioxide atmosphere it reflects sunlight strongly. After the Sun and the Moon, it is the brightest celestial body.

It is the only planet to rotate in reverse direction. On Venus the Sun rises in the west and sets in the east. Venus is visible as the morning and the evening star. The Venusian surface proper is hidden under a thick coat of clouds. Venus is therefore considered the ruler of occult intelligence.

As Ishtar or Ashtaroth, Venus was the goddess of sexual love in Babylon, as Aphrodite in Greece. The Greeks distinguished between the ordinary and the celestial Aphrodite. The first ruled over love between man and woman, the second over homosexual love.

With the Hebrews, the Phoenicians, the Egyptians, and the Indians, Venus was male. With the Indians, Venus (Sanskrit Śukra) is the teacher and physician of the Titans. According to the *Mahābhārata* epic poem, Śukra possessed the elixir of immortality, with which he could raise the dead to new life. Among those who received the elixir were his mother and Kaca, a son of Bṛhaspati (Jupiter), who had fallen in love with Śukra's daughter Jayanti. According to Indian tradition, the planet Śukra has sixteen rays.

Venus is strongly related to alchemy.

This planet rules the arts, harmony, proportion, affection, and the ability to integrate separate things into a whole and to mediate between opposites (sign of Libra). The tendency of Venus is toward cozy relaxation. Venus is likewise strongly related to music.

Venus rules over the metamorphosis of the cells, the reproduction and enrichment of the substances, the formation of tissue, the selection and transformation of substances in the cells, the preservation of the body, the complexion, the relaxation of tissue, the face, the cheeks, the chin, the upper lip, the abdomen, the throat, the kidneys, and the parathyroid glands (which act as intermediaries and stabilizers for the muscles, the formation of nerves, and nervous energy, and decisively influence the calcium metabolism by their hormone), the thymus gland, the stomach veins, the appetite, the breasts, germination, the chyle (chylus) in the intestines, the diuretic and emetic processes, the eustachian tube, exosmosis, fermentation, fertilization, the inner sexual organs, the harmony within the systems, the umbilicus, the neck, the nose, the sense of smell, the palate, and the spine (with the Sun, Mercury, Neptune, and the sign of Leo).

Something has already been said above about the image of Venus (Ishtar-Aphrodite-Śukra). No influence of Venus or Jupiter could in any way promote disease, which is only promoted through critical aspects of other planets. A badly configured Venus promotes diseases of the uterus and the sexual organs as well as of the kidneys. Diseases promoted by intemperance and excesses are Venusian.

Venusian metals and minerals are copper, pink corals, jade, and, according to the Indian tradition, diamonds. The zodiacal signs are Taurus and Libra. Venusian scents are sandalwood, storax (Taurus), and galbanum (Libra).

Plants That Come Especially under the Dominion of Venus

Achillea millefolium: yarrow
Ajuga reptans: bugle
Alchemilla vulgaris: lady's mantle
Alkanna tinctoria: dyer's alkanet
Althaea officinalis: marshmallow
Aquilegia vulgaris: columbine

Arctium lappa: burdock, burr fruit

Artemisia absinthium: wormwood (with Mercury and Mars)

Artemisia vulgaris: mugwort

Betula pendula (= verrucosa): a kind of birch

Betula pubescens (= alba): a kind of birch

Castanea sativa: chestnut (with Jupiter)

Cicer arietinum: chick-pea

Cotyledon umbilicus: navelwort, cotyledon

Cynara scolymus: artichoke

Digitalis purpurea: digitalis, red foxglove (with Mercury and Saturn)

Dipsacus sativus: teasel, fuller's thistle or weed

Fragaria vesca: wood strawberry, wild strawberry (with the Sun and Jupiter)

Geranium robertianum: geranium, herb Robert (with Mars)

Glechoma hedera: ground ivy (with the Sun)

Leonurus cardiaca: motherwort

Lithospermum minus: gromwell

Menthae: all kinds of mint

Meum athamanthicum: spicknel

Nepeta cataria: catnip

Orchis: all kinds of orchids

Oxalis acetosella: wood sorrel, clover sorrel

Persica vulgaris: peach

Phaseolus vulgaris: dwarf bean, running bean (with the Moon)

Primula officinalis: primrose

Prunus cerasus: morello cherry, sour cherry

Pyrus communis: pear

Pyrus malus: apple (with the Sun)

Rosa damascena: rose (with Jupiter)

Rubus fructicosus: blackberry

Rumex acetosa: sorrel

Sambucus nigra: elder (with Saturn and Mercury)

Sanicula europaea: sanicle

Saponaria officinalis: soapwort, soap plant, soapweed

Senecio jacobaea: tansy ragwort
Senecio vulgaris: groundsel
Solidago virga aurea: goldenrod
Thymus serpyllum: wild thyme (with the Sun)
Thymus vulgaris: garden thyme (with the Sun)
Triticum sativum: wheat (with Jupiter)
Verbena officinalis: vervain
Viola odorata: violet (with the Moon)

Therapeutic effects of Venusian plants are alterative, diuretic, anti-nephritic, emollient, emetic, and harmonizing.

♂ Mars

Mars, the first of the outer planets, has two moons, Daimos and Phobos. The red-orange surface of the planet consists mainly of iron and aluminum. In 687 days Mars revolves around the Sun; in 780 days it runs through the zodiac.

The effect of Mars is violent, accelerating, and intensifying. Mars is the active principle, dynamic energy. If well applied, the Martian forces are constructive; if uncontrolled, they result in destruction.

Physiologically, Mars rules the muscular system, the red corpuscles, the body heat, and the combustion processes in the body, the sexual organs, the suprarenal capsules, and, together with the Sun and Jupiter, the formation of blood. From food it absorbs the iron that it transmits to the blood.

The Sun and Mars together bring vitality, initiative, and courage. Mars also shares in the vital processes (with Jupiter and the signs of Leo, Libra, Scorpio, Sagittarius, and Virgo).

Mars also influences the motor nerves, the left half of the brain, the gall, the fibrin in the blood, the rectum, and the astral body.

According to Paracelsus, Mars rules over the polarity between the brain pole (Aries) and the sexual organs (Scorpio), that is, the beginning and end of the serpent power.

Mars further rules over the diaphragm, the left ear, the purging processes, the head and head injuries, inflammations, and surgical treatments.

The image of Mars is male, aggressive, warlike (martial), and intensely sexual, with the so-called animal magnetism.

Diseases associated with Mars are inflammations of all kinds, small-pox, scarlet fever, typhus, high blood pressure, acute pains, rapidly developing fever processes, and hemorrhages.

Martian metals and minerals are iron, steel, cinnabar, ruby, and dark red corals. Martian scents are mustard, garlic, cypress, and sulfur.

Plants That Come Especially under the Dominion of Mars

Allium cepa: common onion

Allium sativum: garlic

Aloe: all kinds of aloe (with Saturn)

Ananas sativus: pineapple

Anemone: anemone

Artemisia absinthium: wormwood (with Venus and Mercury)

Arum maculatum: cuckoopint, wake-robin

Bellis perennis: daisy (with the Moon)

Berberis vulgaris: barberry (with Uranus)

Buxus sempervirens: box

Bryonia dioica: bryony

Cassia obovata: senna

Capsicum: paprika, red pepper, various kinds

Carduus benedictus: avens, blessed thistle

Cochlearia armoracia: horseradish

Coriandrum sativum: coriander (with Venus)

Crataegus oxyacantha: hawthorn (with Saturn)

Genista tinctoria: dyer's broom

Gentiana: gentian (yellow)

Geranium robertianum: geranium, herb Robert (with Venus)

Gratiola officinalis: hedge hyssop

Helichrysum arenarium: everlasting flower, immortelle, goldflower

Humulus lupulus: hop

Lamium album: dead nettle, blind nettle, lamium

Linum usatissimum: flax (with Jupiter and Saturn)

Lonicera caprifolium: honeysuckle, woodbine (with Mercury)

Mezereum: spurge-laurel, mezereon

Nepeta cataria: catnip

Nicotiana tabacum: tobacco

Ocimum basilicum: basil (with Jupiter)

Ononis spinosa: restharrow, thorny harrow

Pinus: pine, all kinds

Plantago major: plantain (with the Sun)

Quercus robur: oak (with Jupiter)

Ranunculus sceleratus: cursed crowfoot, marsh crowfoot (with Venus)

Raphanus sativus: black radish

Rheum palmatum: Chinese rhubarb (with Jupiter)

Rosa canina: dogrose (with Jupiter)

Rubia tinctorum: madder (with Jupiter)

Sabina: savin, red cedar

Sambucus ebulus: dwarf elder

Scilla maritima: sea onion, squill (with Saturn)

Scrophularia nodosa: common figwort, knotty brownwort

Smilax utilis: sarsaparilla

Sinapis: all kinds of mustard

Strychnus nux vomica: poison nut, emetic nut

Tormentilla: tormentil, bloodwort, rootwort (with the Sun)

Urtica dioica: common nettle, stinging nettle (with Pluto)

Urtica urens: small stinging nettle (with Pluto)

The therapeutic effects of Martian plants are aphrodisiac, stimulating, tonic, blood-forming, acting upon the blood vessels.

♃ Jupiter

The orbit of Jupiter lies beyond the asteroid belt. The biggest planet of our solar system consists chiefly of hydrogen and helium, and it contains the major part of the matter in the solar system that was not used for the formation of the Sun. This planet has a very strong magnetic field. Jupiter's thirteen moons make the planet appear like a small solar system.

Jupiter gives energy to the Earth. Especially during a conjunction with the Earth (every 399 days), the solar wind brings energies from the magnetic field of the planet. Jupiter circles around the Sun in eleven years and 315 days. In less than ten hours it rotates around its own axis.

Physiologically, Jupiter rules the liver, the arteries and the circulation, especially the arteries of the abdomen and the legs, the enrichment of the blood through food intake, the fibrin in the blood (with Mars and the sign of Pisces), the subcutaneous fatty tissues, the suprarenal capsules, food intake and assimilation, the spleen and the kidneys, the body's powers of resistance, the carbohydrates, the supply of oxygen to the blood, the formation and reproduction of cells, the conservation of energy, the digestive organs, the feet, the sex organs and their veins, the thighs and the buttocks, the lungs, the ribs, the right ear, the sanguine temperament, the semen, the body's sugar economy, the maintenance of the tissues, and the teeth. Jupiter's influence on the occipital lobe of the hypophysis (pituitary body) regulates the fluid circulation and the growth of the body.

Jupiter has its image as the king of the gods, the religious teacher (its Indian name is Guru), the father, the benefactor disbursing riches, but also as the bon vivant very much out for his own desires and gratifications.

Jovian diseases are all diseases due to immoderation in eating and drinking, bad digestion, too much congestion, impure blood. By itself, Jupiter does not cause any sicknesses, except diseases of the blood, the lungs, the liver, and indirectly also of the heart, caused by bad aspects with other planets. A badly aspected Jupiter also promotes strokes, abscesses, convulsions, as well as cancerous processes in certain cases on account of its hyperexpansivity.

Jovian metals and minerals are tin, lapis lazuli, amethyst, blue sapphire, and, according to Indian tradition, yellow sapphire.

Jovian scents are benzoin, carnations, hyacinth, mastic, violet.

Plants That Come Especially under the Dominion of Jupiter

Acer: maple, sycamore

Aesculus hippocastanum: horse chestnut

Agrimonia eupatoria: agrimony

Agropyron cannium: couch grass, dog grass

Althaea officinalis: marshmallow (with the Sun and Venus)

Amygdalum: almond (with the Sun)

Anagallis arvensis: scarlet pimpernel

Anthriscus cerefolium: garden chervil

Arnica montana: arnica

Asparagus officinalis: asparagus

Avena sativa: oats (with Mercury)

Betonica officinalis: hedge-nettle, stachys, woundwort

Borrago officinalis: borage

Castanea sativa: edible chestnut (with Venus)

Centaurium umbellatum: centaury

Cetraria islandica: Carrageen or Irish moss

Chelidonium majus: celandine (with the Sun)

Cichorium endivia: endive

Cichorium intybus: chicory

Dianthus cariophyllus: carnation

Ficus carica: fig (with Venus)

Foeniculum vulgare: fennel (with Mercury)

Fraxinus excelsior: ash (with the Sun)

Fraxinus ornus: manna, flowering ash

Fumaria officinalis: fumitory

Gentiana lutea: gentian, yellow (with the Sun)

Hepaticae: liverwort, different kinds

Hyoscyamus niger: henbane (with Saturn and Neptune)

Hyssopus officinalis: hyssop (with the Moon and Mars)

Imperatoria: masterwort

Inula campana: elecampane

Jasminum: jasmine

Juniperus communis: juniper (with the Sun and Mercury)

Laurus nobilis: laurel (with the Sun), bay

Lavandula vera: lavender (with the Sun and Mercury)

Linum usitatissimum: flax (with Saturn and Mars)

Liquiritia officinalis (Glycyrrhiza glabra): licorice (with Mercury)

Marchantia polymorpha: a kind of Irish moss, liverwort

Melilotus officinalis: melilot, sweet clover

Melissa officinalis: balm (with the Sun)

Mentha piperita: peppermint (with Venus)

Myristica fragrans: nutmeg (with the Moon) or nutmeg tree

Myrrha: myrrh (with the Sun)

Ocimum basilicum: basil (with Mars)

Olea europaea: olive (with the Sun) or olive tree

Panax ginseng: ginseng

Pimpinella anisum: anise (with Mercury)

Pirus malus: apple tree

Polypodium vulgare: polypody

Populus: all kinds of poplars (with Saturn and the Sun)

Potentilla reptans: cinquefoil

Prunus armeniaca: apricot tree

Pulmonaria officinalis: lungwort (with Mercury)

Quercus robur: oak (with Mars)

Rosa canina: dogrose (with Mars)

Rosa damascena: rose (with Venus)

Rubia tinctorum: madder

Rubus idaeus: raspberry

Rumex acetosa: sorrel

Saccharum officinalis: sugarcane

Salvia officinalis: sage

Santalum album: white sandalwood (with Venus)

Santalum rubrum: red sandalwood (with Venus)

Sempervivum tectorum: sempervivum, houseleek

Smyrnium olusatrum: Alexandrian parsley

Solanum lycopersicum: tomato

Symphytum officinale: comfrey

Tanacetum vulgare: tansy

Taraxacum officinale: dandelion

Tilia europaea: lime tree (with Venus)

Tussilago farfara: coltsfoot (with Mercury)

Vaccinium myrtillus: bilberry

Verbascum thapsiforme: mullein

Viscum album: mistletoe (with the Sun and Moon)

Vitis vinifera: grapewine (with the Sun)

The therapeutic effect of Jovian plants is chiefly stimulating, antispasmodic, soothing, emollient, anthelmintic, hepatic, and influencing the circulation.

♄ *Saturn*

Saturn, almost as big as Jupiter, differs from the other planets because of its rings of thin layers of ice particles. Saturn is cold and dry. Ten moons circle around the planet. In twenty-nine years and 167 days Saturn revolves around the Sun.

As the planet of restriction, limitation, and contraction, it is the opponent of Jupiter, whose expansivity it counterbalances. In the ancient tradition, Saturn has the image of a "bad-luck" planet. Saturn is considered the planet of fate, of *karma;* it is the cosmic bookkeeper. Its influence is "hostile" only for individuals lacking self-control. Self-knowledge and discipline are prerequisites for the positive Saturn influences. Undisciplined persons experience Saturn as a punishing teacher.

Saturn is the sage and the guardian of the threshold to the supernatural. Mythologically, he was the god of time among the Greeks: Chronos, the old man with the sickle. Saturn is also linked with agriculture.

Saturn rules over age and all slow and chronic processes. Physiologically, it dominates all aging processes, the bone structure, the teeth, the spine (with the Sun, Neptune, and the sign of Leo), all hardening processes, the anterior lobe of the pituitary body (which restricts the processes of growth and glandular secretion), crystallization processes, the auditory organs, the left auricle (if Saturn is in Leo), the endocardium, sterility, the bladder, the composition of the blood (with the Sun, Jupiter, Venus, Mars, and the signs of Leo and Aquarius), blood circulation in the tissues, the joints, the calves, the cervical vertebrae (Saturn in Taurus), absorption and assimilation of intestinal fluids, the vagus nerve, minerals in the blood, the gall (with Mars, Mercury, the Moon, and the signs of Leo and Scorpio), the knees, memory, the spleen (with the Sun and the signs of Scorpio and Virgo) and their defensive regulation (diathesis), as well as all contracting processes.

Diseases associated with Saturn are rheumatism, hardenings, calcification, melancholy and depression, chronic diseases, lethargy, frigidity, eccentricity, crankiness, and diseases of the Saturnine organs. Saturnine metals and minerals are lead, onyx, chalcedony, black corals, and the lodestone.

Saturnine scents are benzoin, cypress, poppy, resins, and quince.

Plants That Come Especially under the Dominion of Saturn

Aconitum napellus: aconite, monkshood (with Mars)

Aegopodium podagraria: ashweed, wild masterwort, goatweed, bishop's weed, or herb gerard

Aloe: aloe (with Mars)

Allium cepa: kitchen onion (with Mars and the Moon)

Amaranthus: amaranth

Arctium lappa: bur, burdock (with Venus)

Asplenium: spleenwort

Atropa belladonna: belladonna, deadly nightshade (with Mars)

Auricularia judae: jew's ear

Beta vulgaris: beetroot

Beta rubra: beet, mangel-wurzel, stock beet, silver beet

Cannabis sativa: hemp (with Neptune)

Capsella bursa pastoris: shepherd's purse

Carvum carvi: caraway (with Mercury)

Carvum cari: caraway (with Mercury)

Centaurea cyanus: cornflower, bluebottle, knapweed, bullweed

Centaurea nigra: centaury

Cicuta virosa: cowbane, water hemlock

Conium maculatum: hemlock (with Neptune and Uranus)

Crataegus oxyacantha: hawthorn (with Mars)

Cydonia vulgaris: quince

Digitalis pupurea: digitalis, foxglove (with Mercury and Venus)

Epilobium angustifolium: willow herb

Equisetum arvense: horsetail

Eryngium maritimum: eryngium, sea holly

Eryngium campestre: eryngo (common)

Eryngium planum: flat-leaved eryngo

Fagus silvatica: beech tree

Filix mas (Aspidium filix mas): male fern

Foenum graecum: fenugreek

Fumaria officinalis: fumitory

Gaultheria procumbens: wintergreen

Hedera helix: ivy

Helleborus niger: hellebore, Christmas rose

Hieracium pilosella: hawkweed

Hordeum: barley

Hyoscyamus niger: henbane (with Jupiter and Neptune)

Ilex aquifolium: holly

Iris florentina: Florentine iris (with the Moon)

Iris germanica: German iris (with the Moon), dark blue flowers

Iris pallida: pale iris (with the Moon), dark blue flowers

Linum usitatissimum: flax (with Jupiter and Mars)

Listera ovata: twayblade

Lolium temulentum: bearded darnel, cockle weed

Mandragora officinarum: mandrake (with Mercury and the Moon)

Mespilus germanica: medlar

Osmunda regalis: royal fern (with the Moon)

Papaver rhoeas: corn poppy (with the Moon)

Papaver somniferum: opium poppy (with the Moon)

Pinus sylvestris: Scotch pine

Plantago coronopus: plantain

Plantago psyllium: fleawort

Polygonatum officinale: Solomon's seal

Polygonum vulgare: polypody root

Populus: all kinds of poplars (with Jupiter and the Sun)

Prunus spinosa: sloe, white plum, blackthorn

Rhamnus frangula: alder buckthorn

Sambucus nigra: black elder (with Mercury and Venus)

Scilla maritima: squill, sea onion, (with Mars)

Secale cereale: rye

Senna: senna

Solanum dulcamara: bittersweet nightshade

Sorbus domestica: service or sorb tree

Stellaria media: chickweed

Symphytum officinale: comfrey (with Jupiter)

Tamarindus indica: tamarind

Taxus baccata: yew

Ulmus campestris: elm (with Mercury)

Veratrum album: white hellebore

Verbascum phlomoides: mullein

Verbascum thapsiforme: common (great) mullein

Vinca minor: periwinkle (with the Moon)

Viola tricolor: pansy

Zea mays: maize, Indian corn

The chief effects of Saturnine plants are stimulating, contractive, sedative, coagulant, mineralizing, and bone-forming.

Days, Hours, and Rhythms of the Planets

Every day of the week is ruled by a planet:

> Sunday by the Sun
> Monday by the Moon
> Tuesday by Mars
> Wednesday by Mercury
> Thursday by Jupiter
> Friday by Venus
> Saturday by Saturn

According to our calendar, every day begins at midnight (0 hour) and ends twenty-four hours later at midnight.

In the astrological tradition, this is not necessarily so; there are also other systems. On these systems depends the calculation of the planetary hours. Let us now consider some of these systems.

Practically all traditions agree on the sequence of the planetary hours. The following sequence always applies:

> Sun
> Venus
> Mercury
> Moon
> Saturn
> Jupiter
> Mars

The first hour of a day is in each case ruled by the planet of the day; therefore, the first hour of Sunday by the Sun, the first of Monday by the Moon, and so on. After this first hour the other hours follow in the above-mentioned sequence. After the seventh hour the sequence is repeated. The eighth hour of Sunday is again ruled by the Sun. Opinions agree on this.

The views differ, however, as to which hour is to be considered the first of the day, and also how long a respective planetary hour lasts. We shall now briefly discuss several views.

According to the kabbalistic tradition, the day always begins at dusk, or sunset. Consequently, Saturday begins on Friday evening at sunset and ends on Saturday with sunset.

In the course of time, two systems developed, the fixed and the flexible.

1. According to the kabbalistic system, every day begins at 6:00 P.M. local time and ends the following day, after twenty-four hours, at 6:00 P.M. The accompanying tables represent this system (figures 34 and 34a):

Hours	Sunday	Monday	Tuesday	Wednesday	Thursday	Friday	Saturday
18–19	☉	☽	♂	☿	♃	♀	♄
19–20	♀	♄	☉	☽	♂	☿	♃
20–21	☿	♃	♀	♄	☉	☽	♂
21–22	☽	♂	☿	♃	♀	♄	☉
22–23	♄	☉	☽	♂	☿	♃	♀
23–24	♃	♀	♄	☉	☽	♂	☿
24–1	♂	☿	♃	♀	♄	☉	☽
1–2	☉	☽	♂	☿	♃	♀	♄
2–3	♀	♄	☉	☽	♂	☿	♃
3–4	☿	♃	♀	♄	☉	☽	♂
4–5	☽	♂	☿	♃	♀	♄	☉
5–6	♄	☉	☽	♂	☿	♃	♀

Fig. 34

2. According to the flexible system, instead, the day always begins with the moment of sunset and ends at sunset of the following day. The exact time of the sunset must therefore be known. The sequence of the horary rulers, however, is always the same.

In another view, the day begins, not at dusk, but with the morning hours. Here, too, there are two systems, a fixed and a flexible.

3. According to the fixed system, the day always begins at 6:00 A.M. in the morning and ends twenty-four hours later.

4. According to the flexible system, the day begins with the moment of the sunrise. If, for instance, the sun rises at 5:22 A.M. local time on a Sunday, the time from 5:22 to 6:22 A.M. is the hour of the sun, from 6:22 to 7:22 the hour of Venus, from 7:22 to 8:22 the hour of Mercury, and so on. Monday begins with the Moon hour at the

Hours	Sunday	Monday	Tuesday	Wednesday	Thursday	Friday	Saturday
6–7	♃	♀	♄	☉	☽	♂	☿
7–8	♂	☿	♃	♀	♄	☉	☽
8–9	☉	☽	♂	☿	♃	♀	♄
9–10	♀	♄	☉	☽	♂	☿	♃
10–11	☿	♃	♀	♄	☉	☽	♂
11–12	☽	♂	☿	♃	♀	♄	☉
12–13	♄	☉	☽	♂	☿	♃	♀
13–14	♃	♀	♄	☉	☽	♂	☿
14–15	♂	☿	♃	♀	♄	☉	☽
15–16	☉	☽	♂	☿	♃	♀	♄
16–17	♀	♄	☉	☽	♂	☿	♃
17–18	☿	♃	♀	♄	☉	☽	♂

Fig. 34a

moment of sunrise, followed by the Saturn hour, the Jupiter hour, the Mars hour, the Sun hour, the Venus hour, the Mercury hour, then again a Moon hour, and so on, in the usual sequence.

5. A fifth system divides the day and night halves into twelve "hours" each. As day and night have different lengths in different seasons, the duration of the planetary hours of this movable system varies. In winter, there are twelve short daytime "hours" and twelve long night "hours." The planetary hours of the day are therefore shorter, those of the night longer than sixty minutes. In the summer it is the reverse.

6. A sixth system divides the twenty-four hours of the day into seven even periods and considers these the planetary hours. This way results in planetary hours of approximately three hours and twenty-five minutes' duration. The hour in which sunrise falls is the hour of the planet that rules the respective day. The table in figure 35 illustrates this system.

The last-discussed system is considered the best by many. The calculations are simple and always the same; we are dealing with a fixed system. After this, the systems discussed under (3) and (4) are probably the most popular. Thus, similar to the concept of the zodiac, there are also fixed and flexible systems for the calculation of the planetary hours.

Hours	Sunday	Monday	Tuesday	Wednesday	Thursday	Friday	Saturday
0.00–3.26	♂	☿	♃	♀	♄	☉	☽
3.26–6.52	☉	☽	♂	☿	♃	♀	♄
6.52–10.18	♀	♄	☉	☽	♂	☿	♃
10.18–12.44	☿	♃	♀	♄	☉	☽	♂
12.44–17.10	☽	♂	☿	♃	♀	♄	☉
17.10–20.36	♄	☉	☽	♂	☿	♃	♀
20.36–24.00	♃	♀	♄	☉	☽	♂	☿

Fig. 35

Indian astrology works more with the fixed (sidereal) zodiac, Western astrology schools more with the flexible (tropical).

In conclusion, we shall mention the *tattva* vibrations.

TATTVA	PLANETS
Ākāśa	Saturn
Vāyu	Mercury
Tejas	Sun/Mars
Apasa	Moon/Venus
Pṛthivī	Jupiter

Fig. 36

These are vibrations of the great world ether that oscillate at the rhythm of twenty-four minutes. Four different *tattvas* follow each other, every two hours a complete *tattva* circle ends. Every *tattva* period is ruled by one or two planets. The cycle begins at sunrise. Figure 36 is a representation of this.

Calculations of the planetary hours are always done according to local time, not according to the zone time nationally in effect.

How do we find the exact local time? The process is simple. First we calculate the corresponding Greenwich Mean Time (GMT). It is one hour behind Middle European Time (MET). Thus, 10:00 A.M. in Switzerland corresponds to 9:00 A.M. GMT. Countries with summer time must deduct that, too. For example, 10:00 A.M. in winter in Germany corresponds to 9:00 A.M. GMT, while during summer time it is 8:00 A.M. GMT, since clocks are set one hour ahead in the summer.

After we have found Greenwich time, we must calculate the exact local time. To do this, we must know the exact geographic longitude of the place. For every degree east of Greenwich we must add four minutes to Greenwich time, while for every degree west we must deduct four minutes.

Suppose we wish to calculate the exact local time of Bern, Switzerland, for Tuesday, November 10, 1981, 11:30 MET.

First we reduce to Greenwich time, which would be 10:30 GMT. Bern is located 7°25' east of Greenwich. 7 x 4 = 28; 25 x 4 = 100 = 29 minutes 40 seconds, if we change the 100 seconds into minutes. This time is now added to the Greenwich time we have found:

$$
\begin{array}{r}
10 \text{ hours } 30 \text{ minutes } 00 \text{ seconds} \\
+ \qquad\quad 29 \text{ minutes } 40 \text{ seconds} \\
\hline
10 \text{ hours } 59 \text{ minutes } 40 \text{ seconds}
\end{array}
$$

We have found the true local time, which is 30 minutes and 1 second behind the official time.

Because of the geographic longitude of Bern, the added factor remains constant. For a laboratory in Bern the true local time is therefore always 30 minutes and 20 seconds behind the official time. Consequently, the cycle of the planetary hours begins fully half an hour later.

The time of 11:30 MET, Tuesday, November 10, 1981 (true local time 10 hours 59 minutes 40 seconds) comes under the hour of Venus, if we calculate by the system discussed in paragraph five, since the Venus hour runs from 10 hours 16 minutes (10:16 A.M.) to 1 hour 36 minutes (1:36 P.M.), in round figures.

Why then the knowledge of planetary hours?

The processing of plants takes place on the days and at the hours corresponding to them. Strictly speaking, the work already begins with the gathering of the plants. If, for instance, solar plants are to be processed, Sunday from 3 hours 26 minutes (3:26 A.M.) to 6:51 A.M. (in round figures) would be especially favorable for the beginning and execution of all important works.

A further method for finding the most favorable time in each case is the consideration of the positions of the Moon in the zodiacal signs.

Each zodiacal sign is viewed in connection with a corresponding alchemical work:

♈ Aries with calcination
♉ Taurus with congelation
♊ Gemini with fixation
♋ Cancer with dissolution
♌ Leo with digestion
♍ Virgo with distillation
♎ Libra with sublimation
♏ Scorpio with separation
♐ Sagittarius with incineration
♑ Capricorn with fermentation
♒ Aquarius with multiplication
♓ Pisces with projection

The position of the Moon for each day can be seen in an ephemeris.

If a mixture of plants ruled by different planets is to be processed, the regent of the organ or system for which the medicine is to be especially helpful will be given preference. Thus, for instance, the hour of Saturn for mineralizing medicines for the bone system, the hour of the Sun for cardiac and circulatory remedies, the hour of Mercury for nerve medicaments, and so forth.

Now a few more words about two lunar houses, especially important in alchemy. They play a special role in Oriental alchemy.

According to figure 37, the whole zodiac consists of two halves, a Sun-like or solar half and a Moon-like or lunar half. As we have set the ruling planets in the respective zodiacal signs, the symmetry can easily be recognized: the signs ruled by the same planet face each other.

The path from the sign of Leo to the sign of Capricorn is solar. It is also called the "Dry way." From the Fire sign Leo it leads to the Earth sign Capricorn, which is ruled by Saturn.

Every sign of the zodiac has three decanates of ten degrees each. The lord of the first decanate is always the lord of the whole sign. Thus Saturn in Capricorn, the Sun in Leo. The second decanate (degrees 11–20) is ruled by that planet that rules the next zodiacal sign of the same Element. The Elements of the zodiac are distributed as follows:

Fire: Aries, Leo, Sagittarius
Earth: Taurus, Virgo, Capricorn
Air: Gemini, Libra, Aquarius
Water: Cancer, Libra, Pisces

After Capricorn, the next Earth sign is Taurus, ruled by Venus. Therefore the second decanate of Capricorn is ruled together with Venus. The third decanate of Capricorn, instead, has a tinge of Mercury, since Virgo is the Earth sign corresponding to Mercury.

By this diagram we recognize that the first ten degrees of Capricorn are doubly ruled by Saturn, since both the whole of Capricorn and the first decanate are Saturnine.

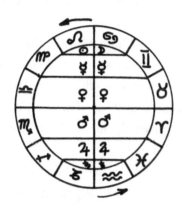

Fig. 37

What is the meaning of all this?

The first ten degrees of Capricorn correspond to doubly Saturnine qualities; consequently, extreme condensation, concretization, crystallization. The position of the Moon in this sign of the zodiac is favorable to the preparation of solid substances, especially the "Stones" so called in alchemy, for which the twenty-second "Moon house" (0°–12°5'26" Capricorn) is promising.

Arabian alchemy and astrology call this Moon house al-Sa'ad al-Dhabid (roughly translatable as "the murder or murderer blessed by good luck"). In other texts this Moon house is also called Caaldalbala or Caalbeba. According to tradition, it is considered propitious for all kinds of healing and for changing enmity into friendship. To pray for the necessary blessing, the Arab alchemist turns to God at this time by revering the divine name of al-Karim (the Gracious one).

How about the other Moon house?

The degrees 21°25'45" to 4°17'10" of Pisces form the twenty-sixth Moon house. It is in this Moon house that the transition from the Saturn sign of Aquarius to the Water sign of Pisces falls, which is ruled by Jupiter (and Neptune). What is solid is volatilized; what is hard becomes subtle and volatile. The whole path from Aquarius to Cancer is called the "Wet way." It begins in the Element Air and ends in the Element Water. This way, and especially the twenty-sixth Moon house, are favorable to the preparation of liquid and volatile substances, that is, the so-called Circulata or Alkahests, which are also called volatile Stones.

The Arabic name of this Moon house is al-Fargh al-Mukdim (upper hole of the udder or tube). Other names are Algafarmuth, Algafarbuchor, Algazaldi, or Alm. According to tradition, this Moon house is favorable for marriage, agriculture, and trade. The corresponding Muslim name of God is al-Latif (the extremely Subtle One), in whose sphere the jinns of the Elements have their tasks.

Finally, we will here mention that Indian alchemy considers the sixth night of the decreasing moon especially favorable for the preparation of alchemical medicines.

The diversity of the horary systems may confuse the reader. Which view is best? That is for each to find out for himself. The views seem to contradict each other, but it is possible that several systems overlap. All systems discussed have their representatives. I am most inclined toward the system discussed in paragraph six, since it continues the natural septenary division of the chronological order. Seven is in a special way the number of chronological time, just as twelve is the number of space. Next to this system, those discussed in paragraphs three and four seem to me the most convincing.

A method beyond this controversy consists in establishing the actual planetary positions in each case, hence the precise horoscope of a point in time, calculated for a certain place. Here now are some explanations concerning this.

The Exact Horoscope as the Basis for the Works

To obtain a complete picture of the stellar influences at a specific moment, it is necessary to cast an exact horoscope, that is, to pinpoint the actual position of the planets. To do this, a knowledge of astrology is required.

Of course, the spagyrist cannot move the planets in conformity with his wishes, but he can await favorable positions; in addition, he can "move" the houses of the horoscope by computing the moment of a specific ascendant, as well as the Medium Coeli. For this purpose he requires the ephemeris of the year under consideration and a table of houses for the latitude concerned.

First the position of the planets is calculated; the exact position of the Moon is later corrected after determining the ascendant. As soon as the position of the planets for the day in question has been marked in, the most favorable ascendant and the Medium Coeli are sought. These should stand in good angles to the planets. First the desired ascendant is entered, then the time is computed according to the table of houses.

In various ways we can now allow the planets concerned stronger influences. For example:

1. The planet is placed in the first house close to the ascendant or the Medium Coeli, due attention being paid to all signs and aspects.
2. The sign (domicile) ruled by the planet or the sign in which the planet is exalted, or at least one of the decanates ruled by him, is chosen as the ascendant. After working out the favorable aspects, the exact degree of ascendancy is determined.
3. The so-called "negative" aspects (squares, oppositions) are avoided, especially those of Saturn.

4. The ascendant, or the Medium Coeli, is calculated in such a way that Saturn is in the eleventh house ("choosing Saturn as a friend").

5. Special attention is to be given to the most favorable aspects between Sun and Moon, the "negative" ones being avoided.

To compute the most favorable position for a certain work, experience is required. The exact horoscope allows a complete survey of all simultaneous planetary influences.

Experience and experiments have proved that there exists indeed a strong influence by the planetary position in effect. To convince himself, the reader is advised to study the results of the research of L. Kolisko and A. Fyfe.

For important works I prefer to cast an exact horoscope and, like Paracelsus, I would advise every spagyrist seriously to take up the study of astrology.

Two examples now follow concerning the application of an exact horoscope for spagyric works.

In January 1978, a nerve tincture had to be prepared on the basis of valerian. Valerian is essentially a Mercurial plant, and Mercury (with Uranus) very strongly rules the nervous system. A favorable influence of Mercury was therefore desirable. I was in Cosenza, Italy, at the time, and after drawing and examining several possibilities, I decided on January 16, 1978, 5 hours 39 minutes (4 hours 39 minutes Greenwich time)—5 hours 44 minutes true local time in Cosenza, since the eastern longitude of the town is 16.15 degrees. Why this choice?

Let us consider the corresponding horoscope (figure 38).

In the first house, near the ascendant of 0.39° Capricorn, is Mercury. The planet receives three "positive" aspects: a trine of Saturn from the sign of Leo and the eighth house, a trine of the moon from Aries and the fourth house, to which is added a quincunx aspect of Mars in Leo from the eighth house.

In opposition to Mercury we find Jupiter, but Jupiter receives three favorable aspects: a sextile of the Moon, a sextile of Saturn, and a trigon

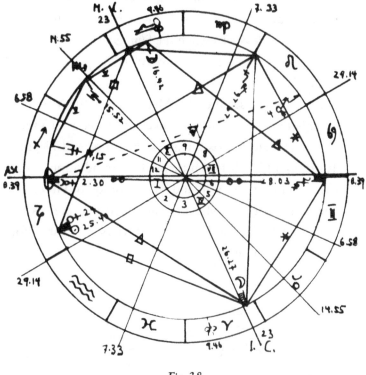

Fig. 38

of Pluto. Uranus is in the eleventh house in a double semisextile aspect to Pluto and Neptune. The three stars Mercury-Saturn-Moon, which form a continuous trine among themselves, irradiate the ascendant intensively.

This is a decidedly strong position.

The situation would be even better without the square between Moon and Sun/Venus and the square of the latter two to the Medium Coeli. Squares have a slowing-down, blocking effect; but we cannot move the stars as we wish. What matters is to make the best of a given situation.

On January 16, 1978, at 5 hours 39 minutes, the 70 percent spirit of wine was poured on the herbs, with which the preparation of the tincture began.

Yet another example. The objective was to find the most favorable moment for a longer and important alchemical work, a magistery requiring several months.

Traditionally, the alchemist starts important works at the time of the New Moon. In the case to be discussed, it was the first New Moon of the natural new year, which begins when the Sun enters Aries.

Here is the horoscope of Saturday, April 8, 1978, 5:22 A.M. in Cosenza (figure 39).

In the first house we see the Sun, Mercury, and the Moon in Aries. In conjunction with the Sun (but not too close) is Venus in Taurus, thus in its own sign. The Sun forms a trine with Saturn and Neptune. The last two also form a trine between themselves. In addition, a quincunx aspect of Uranus falls on the Sun, and an opposition of Pluto.

The conjunction between Mercury and the Moon receives a trine of Saturn, a sextile of Jupiter, and a square of Mars. The latter forms an exact semisextile with Jupiter.

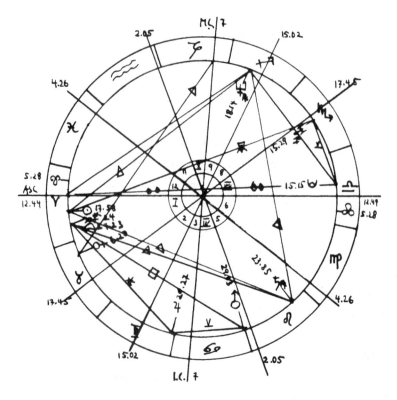

Fig. 39

Venus throws a trine on the Medium Coeli. Uranus and Pluto form a semisextile between themselves.

Sum total: an extremely potent moment at the beginning of the New Moon cycle. Several important works were started simultaneously during this constellation.

In concluding this chapter, let us listen to some advice by Cornelius Agrippa (1486–1535):

Every natural force acts in reality still more wonderfully if, aside from the right physical proportions, it is stimulated and accompanied by attention to celestial things, because lower things must be subordinated to higher things, as woman to man, in order to become fertile.

With every magical operation we must therefore observe the proportions, movements, and aspects of the stars and the planets in their respective signs and degrees, and in what dispositions all these things are in regard to the latitude and longitude of the place, for all that modifies the angles that fall upon the appearance of things with the rays of the celestial bodies. Angles according to which the celestial forces change. Thus, when working with things that stand in relation to a planet, the latter must be exalted, placed and considered in a lucky position and power, to make it lord of the day, the hour, and the aspects of heaven. And not only should the significator of the work be considered, but also how the Moon is turned toward the significator, as nothing can succeed without a favorably positioned moon. If the work requires the ruling of several planets, the stronger ones are chosen, and care has to be taken that they be in favorable aspects; if there are none, the aspects in corner houses are to be chosen. The moment has also to be considered when the Moon has two [aspects], or is in conjunction with one and irradiated by another, or moves from the conjunction or aspect with one [star] into the conjunction or aspect with another. Besides, in the practice of magic Mercury must not be left unheeded, because it is the divine messenger in heaven and on earth, and joined with

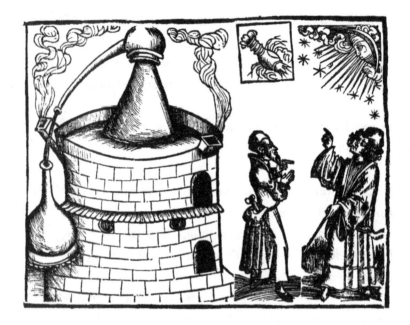

Fig. 40
The Moon in Scorpio during a distillation.

the good planets, it increases their goodness; joined with the bad, it causes the influence of bad luck to grow. A sign or a planet is unfavorable through Saturn or Mars aspects, especially opposition or square, which are inimical aspects, but the conjunction, the trine, and the sextile are favorable aspects. Among these, the conjunction is the most effective, and if the planet is discovered when scrutinizing the trine, it is considered as if it were already in conjunction. All planets, however, fear the conjunction of the Sun and rejoice at its trine or sextile aspects.

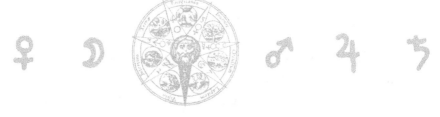

7
PREPARATION OF SPAGYRIC TINCTURES AND ESSENCES

The methods of preparation of spagyric tinctures and essences are varied, although the fundamental principles are always the same. We shall now deal with the most important of these methods.

All spagyric preparations are vehicles of the curative powers of the plants from which they are prepared. Spagyric tinctures and essences are manufactured both as single remedies (simplex remedies) from one plant in each case and as complex remedies from plant mixtures.

Tinctures

We know already that plant tinctures are macerations of plants (or parts thereof) in a dissolving liquid. For the most part, a mixture of water and alcohol is used as a solvent. During maceration the liquid gradually takes on a dark color, hence the designation "tincture," from the Latin *tingo,* "I color." The proportion of dry plants to the liquid varies between 1:5 and 1:10. Frequently, a proportion of 1:8 is used. In all cases we are dealing with proportions by weight.

It is advisable to conform to the regulations in force in each country, and always to keep the proportions constant.

Thus, in the ratio 1:5, for example, 200 grams of dry plants are set to macerate in 1,000 grams of a water-alcohol mixture.

Tinctures can also be extracted from fresh plants. Because of the high water content of the plants used, the alcohol percentage must then be higher, as the water contained in the plants will thin the alcohol. Depending on the amount of the alcohol of the plants used in each case, the exact water-alcohol ratio for the extraction of the tincture must be calculated in advance.

Most of the tinctures are extracted cold or in moderate heat. The temperature must be kept low, especially when using plants containing alkaloids sensitive to heat. On the other hand, tinctures from strongly aromatic plant parts, such as nutmeg, cloves, or cinnamon, are frequently extracted at quite high temperatures, although good tinctures can also be obtained from these through cold-extraction with a sufficiently long time of maceration. Maceration at higher temperatures, for instance at 60° C, are also called digestions.

Percolation and the Soxhlet process represent special extraction techniques. During percolation the solvent is sent slowly, hot or cold, through the plant parts, as in the percolation of coffee. The Soxhlet process is a cyclic percolation, since the extractions are repeated rhythmically.

Most spagyrists work with cold-extractions, or moderate heat (body heat), in the preparation of tinctures. The ancients often macerated in horse dung, which had a gentle, even temperature. The Soxhlet process, which is extraordinarily practical for alchemical work in the mineral world, has but a limited place in plant spagyrics. For the complete extraction of the soluble salts from the calcined plant ash, however, the Soxhlet is very handy, especially as the temperature is then no longer critical.

The Australerba Laboratory in Adelaide extracts part of the tinctures with the help of solar heat. The hermetically sealed extraction tanks are exposed to the heat of the sun for a long time. If the lower part of the tank or the ground on which it stands is of a dark color, it grows much warmer, and a steady rotation of the solvent takes place. In the strong sun of Australia, a dark stone floor that absorbs heat well is sufficient.

When the extracts are ready, the tincture thus obtained is separated from the solid parts, after which the tinctures are sedimented in special tanks, but not percolated. In this way the maximum of valuable components is preserved. With a small spotlight the progressive precipitation of the nonsoluble residue can be controlled from time to time. As the synergistic effect is important with spagyric tinctures, one always tries to take the maximum out of the plants. Maceration times are therefore relatively long. Let us now turn to the processing techniques.

Spagyric Tinctures through Cold-Maceration

In a mixture of water and alcohol—60 to 70 percent alcohol is considered the average rule—the plants are set to macerate according to the selected proportion by weight, for example, 100 grams of plants in 500 grams of 60 percent alcohol. Well suited for maceration is a sufficiently large preserving jar. Its wide neck allows for easily putting in and taking out the herbs, and the rubber ring seals the glass hermetically. The closed glass is now exposed to moderate heat—a place near the radiator or in the sun is well suited. The contents are vigorously shaken at least once every day. Slowly the liquid takes on a dark color. For an ordinary tincture about ten days of maceration are enough.

For spagyric tinctures, we usually extract longer, if necessary up to nine weeks. The tincture then has quite a dark color and a rich, astringent taste.

With a suitable filter we now separate the solid plant parts from the liquid. The plants are thereupon well pressed out once more to obtain the rest of the liquid. This rest is added to the liquid already obtained. The tincture is now filtered through paper, and the residue in the filter paper added to the solid plant parts.

If we are not in a great hurry, we can also free the tincture from the solid components through sedimentation. To do this, we put the tincture into a high glass cylinder that can be closed, or a high flask, and let the solid parts precipitate.

Frequent filtering keeps part of the valuable components back. In addition, part of the essential oils are lost in the process. Therefore, care has to be taken not to "overfilter" the tinctures, which would be equivalent to a fragmentation. Tinctures from resinous-oily plants in particular filter very slowly, although no really impure, solid residue, such as dust, can be recognized.

If we apply the sedimentation process, we finally pour the relatively clear tincture off on top. The precipitated "mud" is then put into a paper filter, and the solid components are thus separated from the rest of the liquid. The rest of the clear liquid obtained in this way is added to the already decanted tincture, and the residue on the filter is added to the solid parts. The tincture is poured into a dark bottle and provisionally put away, well closed. We now have to extract the salts from the solid plant parts. To do this, the remaining plant residues are first completely dried. As our volatile components have already been removed, drying in the sun can now take place. When the plant residues are completely dry, they are burnt to ashes. Well suited for this purpose are the popular flameproof glassware and electric hotplates, or a camping gas burner. Because of the strong formation of smoke, it is better to effect the incineration outdoors. The remaining plant parts cannot simply be set on fire, as they smolder more than burn, and incineration in a flameproof pot has stood the test. The subsequent calcination can then take place in the same container.

Especially well suited for incineration and calcination are the classical wind-furnaces of the ancients. Today, bigger laboratories are using heated combustion furnaces or, as Australerba uses, modern incinerators. They have the advantage that plant residues burn completely without anything added, and a possible chemical contamination by the open gas flame is ruled out. Only at the start of the incineration is a small amount of ethyl alcohol added to set the incineration going. The ethyl alcohol burns completely, the draft then does the rest, and the plants smolder slowly to a pure white ash.*

When the formation of smoke in our flameproof container stops, we have at first some black ash before us—everything has turned to

---

*Small crucible furnaces are also practical. —Ed. of German edition.

charcoal. We now simply heat further toward calcination, and slowly the black ash calcines, gradually changing into white ash. We heat until the ash no longer gets any whiter. There must not be any more black particles of charcoal. Temperatures of 400° to 450° are sufficient for the calcination. A slow calcination at low temperatures is preferable to a short, violent one at high temperatures.

The white ash now contains the soluble salts by which the spagyric tincture is completed. We can add the salts to the tincture in various ways. One way is to add all the ash to the tincture already obtained, shake well, and let the liquid thus extract the soluble salts, while the nonsoluble ones, our Caput Mortuum, sink to the bottom. Shaking daily, we continue extracting in this way up to one week, after which we sediment and pour off the liquid that stands over the precipitate of the Caput Mortuum. The rest is filtered through paper.

Another way consists in extracting the soluble salts from the ash with distilled water, whereby we pour about three times the amount of water on the ash. While stirring, we heat the water just a little. The whole is filtered, and the salt solution thus obtained is then evaporated to dryness. In this way the white salts become visible, and we add them to the tincture.

A third technique consists in extracting the salts with only part of the previously obtained tincture. The tincture containing the salts is then filtered. In this process there is no need to filter all the tincture, which of course means saving time when larger quantities are involved.

After the addition of the salts, the tincture changes color even more. In addition, a change in the aroma can be noticed.

If necessary, the Caput Mortuum can be calcined once again and then added to the tincture so as to extract the rest of the remaining salts. After this, the Caput Mortuum is again precipitated or filtered. Finally, the calcination and extraction of the Caput Mortuum can be repeated yet a third time.

Some spagyrists leave the Caput Mortuum in the tincture, but this method is extremely rare.

We keep the spagyric tincture thus prepared in a dark bottle in a cool place.

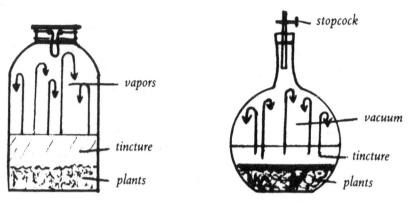

Fig. 41

To take it, a few drops up to a teaspoonful are diluted in water or wine; a cup of lukewarm chamomile tea is also suitable.

If we use a big enough container for the extraction of the plants, good circulation will develop during maceration. The circulation becomes especially intensive if a partial vacuum has been created in the container. To do this, we need a thick-walled flask that can be closed by a rubber stopper with a glass stopcock. We produce the vacuum with a proper pump. Vacuum maceration is gentle but intensive, especially in the sun. (See figure 41.)

Spagyric Tinctures by Soxhlet Extraction

We already know how the Soxhlet Extractor works. With this apparatus we can prepare concentrated tinctures in small amounts in a short time. The dry plants are put into the extraction thimble and slightly pressed against it. The thimble must not be too full if we are to prevent the plants from being washed out during the extraction. We now place the thimble in the extraction chamber of the Soxhlet apparatus and assemble the equipment. On top of the extractor we mount the reflux condenser, through which flows the cooling water. At the bottom of the extractor we attach the flask that contains the solvent. During the first half of the total duration of the extraction process the flask contains nothing but water; the alcohol is added only later. The ratio between the amount of solvent and the plants can be 1:2 or 1:3. In this way we obtain a highly concentrated tincture.

We heat the flask in the sand bath with an electric jacket or directly over a low gas flame. After a short time, the first drops fall into the extraction thimble from the reflux condenser. As long as we continue heating (and cooling the condenser), the surface of the liquid rises steadily until the moment of overflowing. After three or four further overflows, the tincture already has a dark color.

For the second half of the extraction, we now add the necessary amount of alcohol through an appropriate funnel through the tube—open on top—of the condenser. This is followed by three or four alcoholic extractions.

On account of its lower boiling point, the alcohol always evaporates sooner than the water. Consequently, there develops an alcohol cycle. This is the reason we did not add the alcohol at the beginning, as we would then have obtained a predominantly alcoholic extraction. If we wish to effect the extraction from the beginning with a mixture of alcohol and water, the amount of alcohol should not be more than 50 percent of the volume of the extraction chamber of the Soxhlet apparatus.

The alcohol, which at first falls cold into the extraction chamber through the funnel, already starts to dissolve those principles of the plants that the water left behind. We can now clearly see how limited a water extraction is in comparison with a water-alcohol one. Only part of the active principles of the plants are water-soluble. By means of organic solvents, such as alcohol, we obtain the rest of the valuable principles. That is the reason tinctures have been of such great importance from olden times. The ancients also advise maceration in wine or brandy. As these represent a mixture of alcohol and water (aside from other valuable components), the extraction is much more intensive and complete than a simple herb tea or a decoction in water, which always utilizes the plants only partly. An exception is the popular Integral Herbal Elixirs produced by Australerba, which are offered in liquid form as practical herb teas. They are genuine spagyric products, containing the largest possible amount of valuable, active substances. Because of this fact, the teas prepared from them are complete in a special way, hence the name Integral Herbal Elixirs. The methods of production have been developed expressly by Australerba in the course of long research.

For obvious reasons, herbal wines are also especially popular. Already in antiquity we find valuable recipes, for instance the famous cinnamon wine of Hippocrates. Later, the famous distillates are added, which were often developed in monasteries, since knowledge of medicinal plants was particularly cultivated there. But let us return to our Soxhlet apparatus.

After three or four overflows of the tincture, our extraction is finished, and we switch the heater and cooler off. After the cooling, we carefully disassemble everything. The plants are taken from the extraction thimble and dried. Thereafter, they are incinerated and calcined, as previously indicated. Finally, we extract the salts from the ash and add them to the tincture. This process, too, has already been described.

The advantages of the Soxhlet extraction are the concentration of the tincture and the saving of time. Less desirable are the high temperatures, only a little below the boiling point of the solvent. Extractors are also available that work by the cold process, but they require considerably more time if a thick tincture is aimed at. To work with the Soxhlet at low temperatures, we must produce a vacuum at the upper end of the condenser by means of a pump. All connections are made tight with joint grease. Most pumps have a built-in valve and a vacuum meter; if they are missing, we must install them separately. After the extraction of the water is completed, the vacuum must be interrupted for a short time by opening the valve to allow us to add the alcohol. This done, the vacuum is immediately restored.

The Soxhlet process should not be applied too frequently in plant spagyrics. It is useless for plants with alkaloids sensitive to heat, as it simply causes too much loss of valuable principles. A slowly ripening maceration at lower temperatures is preferable in most cases. Not without good reason do the ancients warn us again and again of too-high temperatures and the "vulgar fire."

All tinctures have a limited life span. In time, their therapeutic value diminishes. For at least one year, however, their curative powers remain active, after which their powers decrease slowly. Every spagyric tincture contains considerable curative powers. With sufficient knowledge of botanic medicine we can in this way prepare valuable single and complex remedies.

The prepared tinctures can also be further processed into homeopathic remedies by potentizing them. As their effect thereby turns into a specifically different one, a precise knowledge of homeopathy and spagyrics is therefore necessary. In the meantime, it is advisable to rely on the quality and experience of leading spagyric laboratories. Homeopathic remedies belong in the hands of experienced naturopaths and physicians.

Essences

Essences contain only the volatile constituents of the plants from which they are prepared, since they are always distilled. All solid, nonvolatile components stay behind, except part of the water-soluble salts that are added to the essence at a specific time. Further below, however, we shall see in Glauber's method of preparation that in some cases only the "volatile salts" go into the essences, while the nonvolatile salts stay behind. To word it precisely; the soluble but fixed salts are volatilized in the course of the distillation.

The nature of spagyric essences is subtler than that of spagyric tinctures. They are less "corporeal," more "dematerialized," and their effect is more penetrating, but very subtle. Everything is subtler than with the tinctures. Spagyric essences are therefore considered pure medicines. They are not suitable as household drinks, and they, too, belong in the hands of experienced naturopaths and physicians.

By the processes of potentizing, they can also be turned into highly effective homeopathic medicines. Such medicines are available in pharmacies.

Spagyric essences have a much longer life span—according to experience, a virtually unlimited life span. In many cases the effect even seems to become stronger in the course of time. They ripen like a good wine. For their preparation much experience is required in the art of distilling.

For the preparation of spagyric essences, there are several methods, which we shall now consider separately.

Spagyric Essences Prepared from Tinctures

First we prepare a simple maceration of dry or fresh plants in the normal way in a mixture of water and alcohol as the solvent. Sixty to 70 percent of alcohol is a good average for the solvent.

If the tincture has attained a good color and density after about ten days or more, the whole is carefully distilled. The total content of the maceration container is put as is into a fractionating flask, and a condenser and receiver are attached. It is best to use slow distillation under vacuum at a low temperature in an installation that increases the "expansion factor" (see figure 42).

The empty flask with two joint-connections, inserted between the fractionating flask and the condenser, replaces the classical alembic. It allows for maximum expansion of the vapors, the distance between the molecules becomes great, and the matter is "loosened" (in the alchemistic view). Distillation is finished when the distillate has no more taste. The distillate thus obtained is then stored in a suitable, tightly closed bottle.

Now the total residue in the fractionating flask, including the liquid, is evaporated, or dried, incinerated, and calcined. The solid plant parts can be first separated from the liquid, dried, incinerated, and finally calcined, then the remaining liquid evaporated, the resulting thick condensate carbonized and finally also calcined; or else we can evaporate, carbonize, and calcine the entire residue in a proper flameproof pot without previously separating the solid from the liquid. Now the salts are extracted from the ash with distilled water in the customary manner. The salt solution is then filtered and evaporated, and the salts that have become visible are added to the essence.

As already described above, the white ash can also be directly added

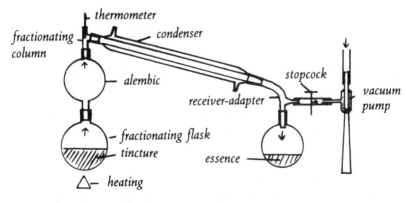

Fig. 42

to the essence after calcination. Thereafter, the essence is shaken every day until it has dissolved almost all the salts out of the ash. After a week, we filter, and the Caput Mortuum that is to be discarded remains in the paper. As indicated before, the Caput Mortuum can be calcined once more and then again added to the essence. After a further week of extracting by daily shaking, we filter again. This process can be repeated a third time. On account of the salts, the otherwise almost colorless essence is colored slightly yellowish. It is stored in a tightly closed bottle. Time will let it ripen further.

Should we prefer fresh or dry plants for the preparation of spagyric remedies? This is a question that cannot be answered as unreservedly as it appears at first.

As we have presumably heard a great deal about the advantage of fresh vegetables and fruit, most of us will probably immediately point to the virtues of fresh plants. On the other hand, the difference in the aroma of a tea infusion of fresh plants and another of dry plants would probably surprise us in many instances. ("Is that really chamomile tea? That has a really grasslike taste, not like the chamomile I know. . . .")

With other plants, the difference will be even greater, for instance, with valerian. During the drying, subtle changes take place in the species, especially in some plants, but those changes are not always to be considered negative.

To be sure, what always matters greatly is the right drying. Good works on botanic medicine provide us with the necessary directions. Mostly, we dry the plants in the shade in an airy place, but many species, and particularly their parts, such as roots, fruits, and so on, can also be dried in the sun or in the stove.

We should not overlook the fact that the great treasure of experience of the botanic medicine has been acquired precisely through the use of dry plants.

Most plants have their "balmy period" in certain seasons, when their curative powers are especially active. Medicinal plants, however, are used the whole year round. The ancients therefore always gathered their plants in the respective seasons. In addition, they also considered the position of the moon and the planets, often also the planetary hours. The plants were then gingerly dried and properly stored, so that they were at all times at hand when needed.

Of course, the use of fresh plants depended strongly on the climate of each country. All "exotic" spices were in any case only available dried. Besides, it was not at all a question of only a few species of plants. If we look through an important classical or baroque herbal, we will be surprised at the precise description and knowledge of "foreign" medicinal plants. How many species of the most distant lands are exactly described there in regard to their curative effects, and how many proven recipes contain "foreign" herbs!

Even today, we buy our herbs mostly in the dried state from the famous herb houses. Herbs gathered at the right time and professionally dried are better than fresh ones gathered at unfavorable times.

On the other hand, fresh plants also have their special advantages because of their own juices, that are still the vehicle of the fullness of the essential vital forces—*provided we pick them at the right moment.* A mere chemical analysis will hardly suffice to "prove" all their active forces. There are energies involved that are on quite different planes. Someone whose consciousness and perception are sufficiently developed to perceive these forces directly can rely on this insight; but not many can do this!

Many distinguished spagyrists, and spagyric manufacturing firms, frequently work with fresh plants, and we also find special directions for the preparation of spagyric essences from fresh plants in the corresponding classical literature. We shall now turn to these methods.

Spagyric Essences from Fresh Plants through Fermentation

As soon as possible after they are gathered, the plants are chopped up and put into a large container. A big preserving jar or a stone pot is well suited. The container must be big enough to prevent any overflowing during the subsequent fermentation. Now a fairly large amount of good, fresh water—spring water is very good—is poured on the plants, and some yeast is added. We cover the container loosely with a lid, and everything is now left to ferment. The time of fermentation differs with the individual plants. The process is complete when the formation of gas ceases.

During fermentation, the alcohol that is forming (*Mercurius in statu nascendi,* i.e., Mercurius in the state of birth) now dissolves the most important principles out of the plants in a very gentle way, while the water absorbs the rest.

After the fermentation is completed, everything is gently distilled, preferably at low temperatures (vacuum!) and in an installation with good possibilities of expansion for the vapors. (See figure 42.)

The ratio between the quantity of the distillate to be expected and the quantity of the medicinal plants used depends on the practice of the individual spagyrist, since no standard regulation exists. As an average practical rule regarding the above-described method, the following may hold good: one part of fresh flowers results in two parts of distillate. To the distillate 15 percent of pure alcohol, preferably pure spirit of wine, is then added.

The entire residue, including the liquid (plant soup) remaining in the fractionating flask, is now evaporated, incinerated, and calcined; we already know the process. From the white ash the salts are extracted as usual. This is done either by adding the ash directly to the essence, filtering the Caput Mortuum off afterward, or by extracting the salts with distilled water. After this, the salt solution is filtered, the salts are made visible by evaporating the water, and they are finally added to the essence. We can repeat the calcination of the Caput Mortuum and the renewed extraction of the salts once or twice. If fresh plants are not available, which can especially happen with exotic plants, the essence can also be prepared from dry plants. In this case, the ratio between dry plants and the quantity of the distillate to be expected is 1:10; that is, 100 grams of dry plants result in one quart of distillate.

Spagyric Essences from Fresh Plants through Fermentation after Addition of Fermentable Sugars

Some spagyrists prefer to add a certain amount of fermentable sugar to the plants to be fermented. In this case, only a small amount of alcohol need be added to the finished essence, as the alcohol content of the distillate is higher. The final alcohol content of the finished essence, however, should never be below 15 percent. Some plants contain only very little sugar. The quantity of alcohol forming can therefore be only quite slight if no sugar is added before fermentation. For the rest, the method of preparation is the same as that already described. As a rule, for the added quantity of sugar the following can be considered valid: 500 grams for 2–3 kilograms of fresh plants.

The plants are chopped up and put into a sufficiently large container. Water, sugar, and yeast are then added, and everything is left to ferment. After the fermentation is completed, the solid is separated from the liquid, and the liquid is filtered and subsequently slowly distilled at low temperatures (possibly under vacuum). When the distillate that has come over becomes insipid, we end the distillation.

The plant residue is dried, incinerated, and calcined. The soluble salts of the calcining material are now extracted with distilled water. We imbibe the ash with about three times the amount of distilled water (estimated spatially in the glass), and heat slightly while stirring. Subsequently, the solution is filtered. The liquid remaining in the fractionating flask is evaporated, the residue is incinerated and calcined, and finally the soluble salts are extracted with distilled water, when three parts of water are taken to one part of ash. After this, the solution is filtered.

The two salt solutions are now poured together and added to the distillate. In so doing, two parts of distillate are taken for one part of the mixed salt solution. If the quantity of the mixed salt solution is greater than half of the distillate obtained, we must reduce it to the desired quantity through evaporation. Nothing must be lost of the salts.

Whoever wishes to obtain the greatest possible quantity of salt can also extract the calcining matter with the Soxhlet Extractor. Since the salts react in an alkaline manner, we can ascertain with litmus paper how far the extraction has progressed.

Spagyric Essences from Fresh Plants with Separation of the Etheric Oils and Subsequent Fermentation of the Residue

In the course of fermentation, heat is released. This leads to a certain loss (though only a small one) of essential oils of the plants used: the oils volatilize. For this reason some spagyrists prefer to separate the essential oils prior to fermentation. We already know how to carry out this separation in the best possible way. (See page 65.) The oils thus obtained are then provisionally kept in a tightly closed bottle.

Drawing off the essential oils at the start of the preparation has still another advantage: the water-plant mixture is sterilized. This will prevent a sudden change in the subsequent fermentation due to undesirable microorganisms.

After separating the oils, the entire residue is fermented with yeast in the fractionating flask. Of course, we wait until the liquid has cooled down to room temperature. After fermentation, we distill gently. The distillation is stopped when the distillate becomes insipid.

We now proceed as usual.

The plant residue is incinerated and calcined, and the salts are extracted with distilled water in the usual manner. The filtered salt solution is then evaporated, and the salts become visible. We store them in a tightly closed glass jar.

In like manner, we now prepare the salts of the fixed Sulfur from the liquid remaining in the fractionating flask. The liquid is evaporated, the residue incinerated and calcined. We extract the salts with distilled water, and the solution is filtered and subsequently evaporated. The salts become visible.

These two salts are now added to the distillate previously obtained. They immediately dissolve in it, and the solution is once again vigorously shaken.

Finally, we still add the essential oils previously extracted, and the whole is once more shaken.

If we wish to work entirely in the classical tradition, we first pour the distillate upon the salts and then let the oil flow into this mixture.

The ancients would say: "The salts are first enlivened (the alcoholic distillate is mercurial = vital principle) and then ensouled (the essential oils of the plants represent the alchemical Sulfur = the soul).

There exists still another variation of the method just described. After the salts have been dissolved in the distillate, this mixture is very slowly distilled at low temperatures. The essential oils are then added to the second distillate. (See also the explanations at the end of this chapter and compare Glauber's instructions below.)

If dry herbs are used instead of fresh ones, they are first chopped up and then macerated for three days in about a sixfold quantity of water.

I prefer maceration in the cold, to prevent possible fermentation. Thereupon, we proceed as described above and begin with the extraction of the essential oils.

Anyone who has carefully read the mode of operation described under this section will have recognized that here an almost complete separation into the alchemical Essentials or Philosophical Principles takes place, since they are made visible individually. For an altogether complete separation, only the rectification of Mercury is missing, that is, the fractionating of the watery-alcoholic distillate.

The Method of Johann Rudolf Glauber

In the second chapter of his famous *Pharmacopoea Spagyrica*, Glauber (1604–1668) describes the preparation of plant essences as follows:[47]

> Take plants with their roots, stalks, leaves, and seed, cleaned of all dirt, at least 50 pounds, as less does not easily ferment, chop it up small, pour water over it, put it into a copper alembic up to a good hand's width, and heat it rather strongly. Now a clear, strongly smelling water goes over with some oil, which is separated in the separator and preserved.
>
> The residue is now taken from the alembic, and fresh herbs are put into it and distilled as before. [The water is distilled together with the essential oil.]
>
> The herbs remaining after the distillation are now imbibed with the distilled water [from which the oil has been removed by the separator], and one or two spoonfuls of young brewer's yeast are added.
>
> Let it ferment in a wooden, covered container for three to four days, until the plants sink to the bottom. In this way it can give off its pure Salt and its volatile Sulfur through distillation.
>
> Now stir the contents of the container well, put everything into the alembic, and distill gently through a condenser, so that the plants do not burn, until a tasteless phlegma comes over; then stop [the distillation].
>
> When now everything spiritual has come over, it is dephlegmatized three times in a row in the water bath with the help of the alembic. [Rectified three times in a row in the water bath with an alembic. See page 74. The alembic allows for a good expansion of the vapors and simultaneously causes a fractionation. To rectify, a fractionating column can also be used. To dephlegmatize means to limit the watery part of the distillate through fractionating, i.e., to rectify the distilled spirit.]
>
> Now the plants are made into bales, which are dried in the sun or near the fire, then burnt to ashes, and from that the Salt is

extracted with its phlegma. [The phlegma is the water that remains after the rectification of the spirit.]

The Salt is made visible through evaporation, then dissolved once more in fresh water, and again made visible; then it is pure.

On one part of the Salt two parts of rectified spirit are poured, and everything is gently distilled in the water bath. Now the spirit attracts to itself as much of the fixed Salt as is necessary, and takes it over with itself, while the fixed Salt retains the phlegma. [Part of the fixed Salt becomes volatile and goes over with the spirit in a gentle distillation, the rest of the Salts retains the rest of the remaining wateriness in the fractionating flask.] The Salt calcined anew [in the fractionating flask] is as good as before. [After evaporating the wateriness, the Salt that stays back in the fractionating flask can be made visible. This Salt is as good as the previous one. The process can be repeated.]

To the quite subtly concentrated spirit [the spirit is simultaneously subtle and concentrated], now pour half of a third of the previously separated oil, shake well, and the spirit immediately dissolves it, and it thereby turns into a clear, strong, and delicious essence, in which the volatile Sulfur of the plants is united with the fixed Salt. [This sentence proves that the Salt that remained in the fractionating flask and which did not become volatile, goes into the essence. We are therefore adding it. The essence contains both the volatile and the fixed Salt. Other masters propose to volatilize part of the Salt through circulation. We shall return to this technique in the following chapter.]

This essence mixes well with all liquids. Because of their subtle purity, a few drops have a rapid effect on all diseases against which the plant [used] is helpful.

For dry plants Glauber recommends a digestion (maceration in heat) of three or four days. The quantitative relation between dry plants and water is 1:6.

I prefer a cold maceration, to prevent possible fermentation. In the event that alcohol should form, the essential oils can no longer be extracted pure, since they are soluble in alcohol.

It is strange that Glauber does not mention the Salts of the fixed Sulfur in his method. Presumably, so little liquid remains after distillation that it is completely absorbed by the plants. The special reference to the burning seems to indicate it. It is also possible, however, that Glauber deliberately withholds the preparation of the Salt of the fixed Sulfur. Such deliberate omissions, as often also deliberate misrepresentations, are not at all rare in the alchemistic literature.

Leaving out the Salts of the Fixed Sulfur seems to me to be a sin of omission. One has but to realize how many valuable components the liquid in the fractionating flask contains after the distillation. Technically, we are indeed dealing with a decoction of the plants. For a true, integral preparation, pouring off this decoction is not advisable.

Finally, we would still mention that distillations are best carried out in the water bath, as it totally excludes burning.

The attentive reader will have noticed that Glauber's mode of operation is closely related to the method described under the previous section

What then have all the methods described in common?

All preparations always contain the three Philosophical Principles, Mercury, Sulfur, and Salt. These Principles were extracted, purified, and then reassembled.

In some instances, Mercury and volatile Sulfur are not separated from each other; only the Salts are first separated and then purified through slow calcination, as, for instance, in the case of tinctures and essences described under sections "Spagyric Essences Prepared from Tinctures," "Spagyric Essences from Fresh Plants through Fermentation," and "Spagyric Essences from Fresh Plants through Fermentation after addition of Fermentable Sugars." In other cases, all three Essentials are separated from each other, for example, by the methods described in this and the previous sections, which begin with the extraction of the essential oils, that is, the volatile Sulfur.

Now a brief remark concerning the second distillation of the "mineralized" Mercury. We have seen by the methods in this and the previous section that the Salts are added to the distillate and that this mineralized spirit is then once again gently distilled. Glauber explains that the spirit absorbs "as much as is necessary" of the fixed Salt and carries it over in the distillation. This at first mineralized and then distilled spirit is also called "Glauber essence."

The distillation of the Salts is of the greatest importance in advanced alchemical works. The so-called volatilization of certain normally non-distillable Salts is one of the secrets that form part of the Great Work. Here, too, several ways lead to the goal; frequent cohobations probably represent the simplest method. (See chapter 10, on the Circulatum Minus.)

Cohobation consists in the renewed distillation of a liquid that has been poured back over the same substance from which it has been extracted through distillation. These distillations are often repeated twenty or fifty times and more! In the alchemistic view, the substance is thus "loosened," "opened," or "exalted." In a similar sense, the circulation is used, also called rotation. We shall deal with it in the following chapter.

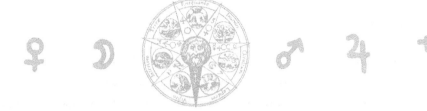

8
CIRCULATION

Circulation, also called rotation or pelicanization, is a specifically alchemistic technique. It represents a form of elevation (exaltatio), which, in the alchemical view, increases the curative power of the essence considerably.

Exaltation is a process whereby a preparation is brought to a higher (subtler) plane of the matter and to a higher energy. (See figures 1 and 2.)

The principle of circulation consists either in a continuous evaporation with a reflux system or in a rhythmization of the essence. In this process a period of expansion and reflux through heating alternates with a period of concentration and calm through cooling. We can therefore speak of a continuous circulation and a rhythmic circulation.

How are these techniques applied?

On the flask containing the essence, we mount a reflux condenser through which the cooling water flows; the flask is then heated (figure 43A). After some time, the volatilizing vapors are condensed in the condenser and fall back into the flask as drops. This rotation remains constant as long as the flask is heated and the cooling water flows. An intensive condenser is best suited for this operation.

We can also put an expansion flask (alembic) between the flask and the condenser. (See figure 43B.)

Circulation can also be carried out under a vacuum, in which case the temperatures remain low. Rotation should always proceed gently and not too violently. If we wish to apply the technique of rhythmic circulation, we switch the heating off after a few hours and let the matter cool; after a few more hours, we heat again. Frequently, circulation is done during the day, while cooling is done at night. This process is repeated seven times, therefore extended over a week. It would then be called a sevenfold circulation. The two side arms of the pelican (figure 44) allow the reflux of the condensate into the lower belly of the vessel, while the upper belly provides space for the expansion of the vapors.

In warm countries, the rotation can easily be done in the sun. If we wish to rhythmize, we put the circulation vessel in the refrigerator overnight.

With a pump over a suitable glass tube with a stopcock, a vacuum

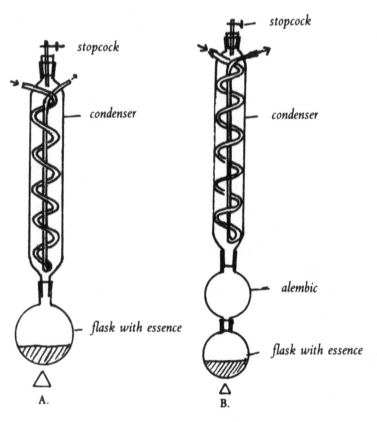

Fig. 43

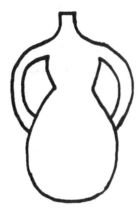

Fig. 44
The pelican. The ancients often used the pelican for circulation.

can be produced, which also results in a good rotation at low temperatures. Figure 45 presents some proposals for fabricating modern circulation containers. Of course, we can also have a classical pelican made by a glassblower.

Until today science has been unable to explain why circulation, especially rhythmic circulation, causes an exaltation of the product. It is similar with homeopathic potencies. Experience proves their validity again and again, but an explanation is beyond the present state of official science. Homeopathy, too, applies rhythmization in its own way,

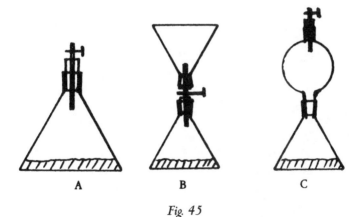

Fig. 45

for instance in succession and also the successive steps of potentizing.

With potentizing, the matter proper decreases while the energy increases; by contrast, with circulation, the quantity of the matter remains constant. For some preparations circulation is a must, for without its application certain preparations would be incomplete.

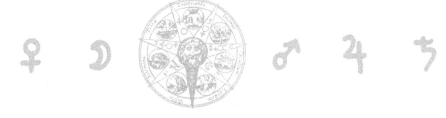

9
THE PLANT MAGISTERY OF PARACELSUS

In his *Book of the Archidoxes,* under the chapter "De Magisteriis," Paracelsus (1493–1541) gives the following directions:

> But the herbs and their likes are to be taken first and mixed with burnt wine and putrefied therewith for one month. After that, distill *per balneum,* and again add more and proceed as before, until there is four times less burnt wine than juice of the herbs. Distill this *per balneum* for one month with new additives; after that separate it, and you will have the magistery of any herb you wish.

This extremely brief text is by no means unambiguous. We should therefore not be surprised that it has been very differently interpreted. Many spagyrists refer to this passage. Let us examine it closely.

The plants are first to be mixed with "burnt wine," which indicates brandy (or spirits), and then "putrefied" therein for one month.

The word *putrefied* here means extracted with alcohol and does not at all refer to decaying, as alcohol makes putrefaction impossible. Through extraction the plants are mutilated in their being; only their "body" remains after extraction. Hence the term *putrefied* implies decomposition, as valuable principles are dissolved.

Paracelsus gives us no quantitative data. Moreover, he does not say whether "month" here refers to a calendar month, that is, thirty days, or a Philosophical Month of forty days. In the alchemical practice, in connection with maceration over a longer period of time, the period of forty days, the Philosophical Month, is frequently applied. Forty is related to darkness; it is the number of waiting and preparation, and hence characteristic of natural processes of disintegration. (For forty days it was raining at the Flood, forty days was the time Jacob's embalming lasted, for forty years Moses led the Israelites through the desert, for forty days Jesus remained in the desert before appearing to the people, and for an additional forty days between Easter and Ascension Day he stayed with his disciples. For forty days Moses stayed on Mount Sinai to receive the Commandments. Indian musicians occasionally undergo a strict yoga-like training period during which they impose certain restrictions upon themselves. The longest of these periods lasts forty days. During this time the musician is not allowed to see the sun.)

After this, everything is to be distilled in the water bath. The distillate contains alcohol, the essential oils, and the water of the plants, together with other volatile components.

"Again add more and proceed as before" means that we add more plants to the distillate obtained and again extract for one month. Subsequently, the liquid is once more distilled in the water bath.

As the plants added to the distillate contain juice, the alcohol content is already thinned in the second distillation, because the major part of the plants' wateriness goes over in the distillation.

We repeat the process of the extraction of new, fresh plants in the distillate, which steadily increases in volume till the alcohol content is one-fifth of the total distilled liquid, that is four times less than the juice of the plants.

If, for instance, we have used 100 milliliters of alcohol for our extraction, fresh plants are successively distilled in the single rounds until the water distilled from the plants amounts to 400 ml and the distillate as a whole amounts to 500 ml. Supposing we used plants with an 85 percent water content, we would then need at least 460 grams of fresh plants for

100 ml of highly rectified alcohol *(vinum ardens);* but as a total distillation of the water from the plants is technically very difficult, we would require up to 600 grams of fresh plants. The one-fifth of alcohol in the final distillate is enough to stabilize it.

Such distilled herb waters were quite in use in the classical pharmacology. Many old works deal thoroughly with both their preparation and their application.[48]

Our distillate now contains all the components of the total quantity of the plants. We are now to circulate (continuously distill) this distillate for one month with *"newen additamentis."*

What additives are meant by these *newen additamentis?* Here now we have a parting of the ways. This so-often-quoted, vague passage of the Paracelsus text has already sparked many a dispute among spagyrists. Everyone knows of it, no one seems to be quite sure of its meaning, and all seem to refer to it. That is how it is with many passages in the classical alchemical literature.

I shall now try to explain my understanding of the famous text, without, however, intending to raise it to a dogma. Presumably, here, too, several ways will lead to the goal.

Anyone who studies the sixth book of the *Archidoxes* attentively can find the way. In it, Paracelsus speaks several times of the so-called Circulata. These Circulata, of which there are higher and lower ones, have the power to extract magisteries from fundamental substances. If now we add an appropriate Circulatum to our distillate, the latter will separate an oily substance that is the magistery proper.

Paracelsus says that one part of this magistery has the same effect as the two-hundredfold quantity of corresponding dry plants (the plant body). (One-half ounce corresponds to 100 ounces.)

According to the specific weight of the fluids, the magistery finally either floats on the surface of the liquids or collects at the bottom of the vessel. Depending on the kind of Circulatum used, the separation proceeds faster or more slowly. At first, a milky cloudiness usually forms, the sign of an emulsion. Later, the droplets collect into an oily mass, and the liquid becomes clear.

In the following chapter we shall speak about a particularly fast-working Circulatum, the famous Circulatum Minus of Urbigerus, which separates within a few minutes. The Circulata mentioned in the *Archidoxes* work more slowly. Because of their ability to separate, the Circulata are also called "liquid Stones" or "the Wet Work." The preparation of the Circulata belongs to the most interesting and surely also the most impressive experiments of alchemy. Therefore, every earnest student should first make an attempt at mastering this difficult "Lesser Work."

After the addition of the Circulatum, Paracelsus now proposes a one-month circulation. The magistery that develops is then separated, for example, with a pipette.

Let us now turn to the Circulatum of Urbigerus.

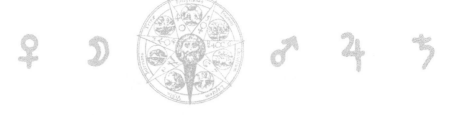

10
THE CIRCULATUM MINUS
OF URBIGERUS

I n the year 1690, there appeared a remarkable publication on the
Circulatum Minus by Baron Urbigerus, which was printed in London by Henry Fairborne. In 1691, a German edition followed, printed
by Johann Caspar Birckner in Erfurt. This edition was followed in
1705 by a reprint in Hamburg by Benjamin Schiller.

The original English title reads: "Circulatum Minus Urbigeranum,
or the Philosophical Elixir of Vegetables with the Three Certain Ways of
Preparing It, Fully and Clearly Set Forth in One and Thirty Aphorisms
by Baron Urbigerus, a Servant of God in the Kingdom of Nature."

The German title mentions, "Still Three Other Ways of Preparing
the Vegetable Elixir Based on Personal Experience. By Baron Urbigerus,
God's Faithful Servant in the Temple of Nature." The linking of his own
name with the Circulatum Minus proves that the Baron considered the
three ways of preparation described as original and entirely his own
contributions.

The actual text consists of a dedication to all serious souls and lovers
of hermetic philosophy, a copper plate, the thirty-one aphorisms, and an
appendix that is a commentary on the copper plate.

What is a Circulatum?

According to the German alchemist Andreas Libavius (1555–1610),

Circulatum means "the Exaltation of a pure liquor [liquid] through a circulating [continuous] dissolution and coagulation in the pelican with heat as the agent."[49]

In the preceding chapter, we said that circulation is an improvement of liquid substances. The liquids are continuously, over a longer time, brought from the liquid to the gaseous state, only to return immediately to the liquid state. Several techniques are united in the art of circulation, which can interconnect digestion, sublimation, distillation, and cohobation.

Digestion means a ripening in mild "digestive" heat by which a substance releases and yields its inner forces. Maceration in warm temperatures is also called digestion. Through digestion thick liquids become subtler, their crude state is modified, and what had been opaque becomes transparent. The impurities, which settle at the bottom, can then be separated. In warmer zones, digestion in the sun is also possible. The ancients often digested in horse dung, which also has a warm, constant temperature in winter. The duration of the digestion is quite variable; it may be a few days, a Philosophical Month, and even longer.

In the course of a *sublimation*, a substance is driven into the upper part of a container by heat and precipitated there.

Distillation separates volatile, or liquid, substances from nonvolatile (solid or fixed) ones, and also different liquids from each other if they have different boiling points and the temperature can be controlled exactly. Continued separation through repeated distillations is called *rectification*.

Rotation and cohobation are related to circulation. The term *rotation* is also used in the same sense as *circulation*. Rhythmic circulation in particular is called rotation.

Cohobation consists of a series of repeated distillations of a solvent over the same substance or the same substances that had been dissolved in it. After each distillation, the distillate is poured back over the residue in the fractionating flask and again distilled, which, according to alchemical concepts, leads to a "loosening" and volatilization of certain materials. To the alchemist it is less important that in this process certain chemical changes occur, since "the same" substances can appear in various forms. (See the remarks about the volatilization of tartar on page 49ff.)

The technique of cohobation is very frequently used in alchemy, and Urbigerus also proposes it for his Circulatum Minus as the actual circulation. (See aphorisms XIV and XV.)

Finally, we should also know that the term *Circulatum Minus* in alchemy can simply mean the alchemical work in the plant world.

In a wider sense, *Circulata* may also stand for the "Aqua Solvens" of Paracelsus, the "Secret Spiritus Vini" of Raymundus Lullus and the Adepts, of "Aqua Mercurialis," the "Spiritus Mercurii Universalis," and others.

Let us now turn to the preparation of the Circulatum Minus of Urbigerus.*

Circulatum Minus Urbigeranum or the Philosophical Elixir from the Vegetable Kingdom, Prepared in Three Different Ways

I

Our Circulatum minus is only a specificated Elixir, belonging to the Vegetable Kingdom, by which without any Fire, or further Preparation of the Vegetables, we can in a Moment extract their true Essence, containing their Virtue, Quality, and Property: which is a great Chymical Curiosity, performing Wonders in the Practice of Physick, and in demonstrating some Works of Nature.

II

We call it Circulatum, because, tho ever so often used in any Extraction, or Chymical Experiment what-ever, it loses nothing

---

*The translations of Urbigerus's aphorisms are from Frater Albertus, *Golden Manuscripts* (Salt Lake City, Utah: Para Publishing Co., 1973). —Ed. of English edition.

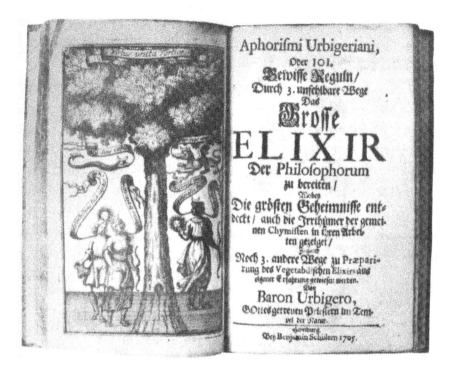

Fig. 46

of its Quality, or Property: which is a Prerogative, pertaining to the Universal Elixir, called also the Circulatum majus, because it commands in all the three Kingdoms of Nature; whilst this, being restrained to one only Kingdom, is for that reason called Minus.

In alchemy, a difference is made between the Circulatum Minus and the Circulatum Majus. The first is an elixir that can effect in the plant world what the Circulatum Majus can effect in all three kingdoms (plant, mineral, and animal worlds): the separation.

The Circulatum Minus, provided it is prepared in the right way, loses nothing of its vigor even after frequent use. A Circulatum Minus that I prepared in my Italian laboratory many years ago still separates today within a few minutes. After every separation the Circulatum Minus can be recovered through a gentle distillation. We shall see further below how to do it.

III

Out of Diana's undetermined Tears, when Appollo has appeared, after the Separation of the three Elements, Determination, Digestion and glorious Resurrection, we can, without the Addition of any other created thing, prepare this our determined Elixir: Which is the first, noblest, and secretest way of the Philosophers.

The "Tears of Diana" are the pure Mercury, the ethyl alcohol not yet specified by any kind of additives. Later it is determined by the addition of the Salts and essential oils.

"When Apollo has appeared" means after the volatile Sulfur—that is, the essential oils—has been distilled from the plants. The appearance of Apollo, which is the separation of the essential oils, is always the first step in separation.

Urbigerus writes that the separation of a species into its three Essentials or Philosophical Principles (here called the Elements) is always a prerequisite for the work. The Mercury is then "determined" by the addition of the other purified Principles, that is, the Salts, the fixed and the volatile Sulfur. This is followed by a digestion with subsequent distillations (cohobations). In this way we can prepare the Circulatum Minus from a species without any additives. Urbigerus considers this the noblest way.

IV

The Determination of our Diana's Tears consists only in their perfect and indissoluble Union with the fixt Vegetable Earth, philosophically prepared, purified, and spiritualized: for the love of which they are forced to leave their first universal undetermined Property, and be clothed with a determined particular one, which is required to this our Circulatum Minus.

Urbigerus explains clearly what he means by the determination of Diana's Tears. But the Salt (fixed vegetable earth) obtained from the plant body (the plant residue) through calcination must be prepared "philosophically," that is, in the proper alchemical way, therefore correctly calcined, purified, and spiritualized (volatilized). In the course of this treatment, the nature of the Salt is changed.

V

Our second way of preparing this our Vegetable Elixir is by a right Manipulation of a Plant of the noblest Degree, standing by itself, or supported by others: after the Preparation of which, and its Putrefaction, Reduction into an Oil, Separation of the three Principles, with their Purification, Union, and Spiritualization, the whole is to be turned into a spiritual ever-living Fountain, renewing every Plant, that shall be plunged into it.

Urbigerus here refers to the wine. During the alchemical work with wine, known as *Opus Vini,* the moment comes when the alchemist can choose between the preparation of a volatile liquid or a solid result, a so-called "Stone." In alchemistic parlance, we would say he can choose the "Wet Way" or the "Dry Way." To understand the term "to become oil," a passage from Glauber is quoted here:

The process of preparing one's oil from wine and of bringing it to a cordial and delicious essence through its own Sal fix and volat. Here I do not refer to the evil-smelling distilled ∴ from ♄ or dregs of wine, but a delicious, pleasant, light, and clear one.

In the fall, when the grapes are pressed, do not let any separate impurities of grape skins or anything else get into the must. Let it ferment in a barrel until it is white, still half-sweet, and most of the feces have settled: N.B.: If you do it earlier or later, then something goes wrong with the ∴; either the must has not yet let go of it or the ∴ has already fallen to the bottom with the dregs. Therefore, watch the time. Then distill the —⌃— out of a ♃-plated ♀ alembic; there will not be much of it. When no more Spirit goes over, remove the cap and pour the residue into clean glasses. Let it stand several days; then a white ∴ will form on top and sometimes precipitate, which should be separated from the must and used for the above-mentioned essence. The must, from which the ∴ and ⏷ have been separated, is added to other must, fermented anew, and it again turns into wine. If you do not know what to do with it, make ⌗ of it. N.B.: There will not be much ∴, which, however, is the best part, just as in all plants. This essence is an antidote, because no venomous animal can stay in the grapes during the time when the vine is in blossom. N.B.: The Essences must be preserved with double bladders and not with wax, which would melt. Put 1, 2, 3, or more fluidrams of herb essence into a jar of wine, shake well, and you will thus obtain a clear, delicious herb wine, so that various wines can be drawn from a barrel by means of various essences. And herewith this First Part is finished. Honor be to God alone!

For the Opus Vini, we would also mention two texts:

1. *Tractatus de Quinta Essentia Vini, in Eröffnete Geheimnisse des Steins der Weisen oder Schatzkammer der Alchymie* (Graz, 1976), pp. 322–35.
2. Johannes Isaaci Hollandi, *Opera Vegetabilia, in Sammlung unterschiedlich bewährter Chymischer Schriften* (Vienna, 1773), pp. 197–304.

The whole process is too long to be described here. We shall later hear something about the so-called Stones. But first to continue with the Circulatum Minus, we shall concentrate on the first and the third ways.

VI

The third and common way is only a Conjunction of a fixt Vegetable Salt with its own volatil sulphureous Spirit, both to be found ready prepared by any vulgar Chymist, and since in their Preparation the purest Sulphur, containing the Soul, has suffered some Detriment by their not being philosophically manipulated, they cannot be inseparably joined without a sulphureous Medium, by which the Soul being strengthened, the Body and Spirit are also through it made capable of a perfect Union.

The conjunction of a fixed plant salt, which we obtain from the plant body through calcination and subsequent extraction of the ash and purification through repeated dissolution and evaporation, with its own sulfurous spirit leads to our Circulatum. The "volatile sulphureous Spirit" is an alcoholic essence distilled from a plant species. "Sulphureous Spirit" always means an alcoholic distillate that contains the essential oil (i.e., the volatile Sulfur) of the plant in question.

These aromatic essences were also frequently made by common "chymicis," that is, by ordinary pharmacists who did not master the spagyric art. The latter are also considered "chymici hermetici" in contrast to the "common chymicis." Examples of the above-mentioned aromatic essences are the well-known "Carmelite Water," even today popular under the name Klosterfrau Melissengeist, and the "Hungarian Water" or "Water of Elizabeth of Hungary," which was also sold as a cosmetic.

These waters of sulfurous spirits are distillates. They do not contain the fixed part of the Sulfur or its Salt, as they did not go over in distilling because of their fixed nature and were therefore discarded. From the alchemical viewpoint, this fractionating is unphilosophical, since the fixed Sulfur contains the other part of the soul. We shall see later that the organic acids that the fixed Sulfur contains are the key to the secret of the volatilization of the Salts. Since the organic acids contained in the distillate called sulfurous spirit do not suffice, others have to be added from outside. Then they act as catalysts and bring body (Salt) and spirit (Mercury) together.

In the following aphorism Urbigerus tells us what this sulfurous matter is and where we can obtain it.

VII

The proper Medium, requisite for the indissoluble Union of these two Subjects, is only a sulphureous and bituminous Matter, issuing out of a plant, living or dead, which is to be found in several parts of the World, and is known to all manner of sea fishermen (the Copavian we find to be the best, and after that the Italian), by which, after it has been separated from its feculent parts through our Universal Menstruum, all the Pores and Atoms of the fixt Vegetable Salt, which is extremely fortified by it, being dilated, it is made capable of receiving its own Spirit, and uniting itself with it.

Urbigerus here clearly refers to resins. These are complex mixtures mainly of aromatic substances with properties of acids, besides alcohols, phenols, strongly unsaturated substances. Resins are closely related to terpenes. We obtain resins by injuring certain trees, especially pines (spruce), firs, larches, and other exotic trees.

A special resin is amber. Urbigerus's text contains a decisive pointer: "and is known to all manner of sea fishermen." This obvious reference to amber put the author on the right track. Succinic acid (acid of amber) is an excellent catalyst.

But Urbigerus himself tells us which kind of resins he considers particularly suitable for the work.

First he mentions the Copavian, which is Copaiva balsam obtained from *Copaiva balsama*. He considers this best. Next he recommends Italian resin. This is either the resin from the pines widespread in Italy, which give the landscape its characteristic look, or of the cypresses that are also typical of the Italian landscape. Pines are often mentioned in Italian poetry, and Ottorino Respighi even wrote a musical piece about them, "The Pines of Rome." On the other hand, I would like to mention that in Italy I was successful with a particularly high-grade Circulatum Minus from cypress. On whichever resin we may decide, it must first be purified of its feculant parts. Distillation would be the best method. In his *Chymischer Handleiter* the seventeenth-century spagyric pharmacist Le Febure describes this process as follows:

How to Distill the Resin Elemi

What is called Gum-Elemi (olive-tree resin) by grocers is resin that comes from a kind of cedar which grows in North Africa. The best kind is whitish, clear, and mixed with some small yellowish parts. Formed into a mass or lump, it gives off a not unpleasant smell when lighted. Some elemi must be pulverized, mixed with three parts of crushed bricks and one part of common salt previously completely dried by heating. Everything is put together into a retort, which is put in a closed reverberating furnace on a reversed earthenware stand with sand; a good receiver is put in front, the furnace is covered, then heated *per gradus* till nothing rises any longer. Part of this oil can be preserved without rectification, while the other must be mixed with three times as much common salt. This mixture is to be put into a glass retort, and the oil is rectified in sand or distilled once more.

For us it is simplest to buy readily clarified resin, be it Copaiva balsam or Canada balsam. Balsams are mixtures of resins and essential oils, partly with aromatic acids. Canada balsam is obtained from the North American balsam fir *(Abies balsamea)*. Strictly speaking, Canada balsam is a turpentine. It contains about 24 percent essential oil, 60 percent resin soluble in alcohol, and 16 percent resin soluble in ether.

I experimented with several kinds of resins when making my Circulata. Since I obtained especially good results with Canada balsam, I would like to recommend it in particular. Even today Canada balsam is used in microscopy and is available in an already filtered, pure form, although it is not exactly the cheapest kind of resin. In Australia, I also had good results with cedarwood oil. If you look carefully at the copper plate in figure 46, you will notice a hole in the tree from which resin flows. The river into which Apollo and Diana step is resinous. On the other side of the tree Diana comes out of the river. She now holds Apollo's sun in her left (receiving) hand—Apollo and Diana have become one being.

VIII

To fortify the Sulphur, and open the Pores of the Salt, no other Method is to be used, but to imbibe the same with the bituminous Matter in a moderate digestive Heat, as if one would hatch Chickens, and as the

Salt grows dry, the Imbibitions are to be repeated, until you find it so fully saturated that it refuses to imbibe any more of the Matter.

"To fortify the Sulphur" indicates that the Salt and part of the Sulfur have already been put together, as one could otherwise not speak of a fortification. Only that which is already present can be fortified. Only the fixed part of the Sulfur is missing, that part that was lost through unphilosophical manipulation. (See aphorism VI.) The volatile part of the Sulfur, that is, the essential oils, are already together with the Salt. We now add the resinous matter, imbibing our mixture of Sal and volatile Sulfur with it. The mixture is then placed in moderate heat, about 40°. Whenever the matter becomes dry, we repeat the imbibition.

IX

In the Course of Imbibitions the whole Mass is at least nine or ten times a day to be stirr'd with a Spatula, or some other Instrument of dry Wood, by which reiterated Motion, the bituminous Matter receives a better ingress into the Body, and perfects its Operation the sooner.

X

Great care is to be taken, that in the performance of the Imbibitions, no kind of Soil or Dust fall into your Matter, for the prevention of which your Vessel may be kept covered with a Paper, prickt full of holes, or any other suitable Covering, and that nothing come near it, which has its own internal Sulphur: for the Pores of the Salt being very much dilated and opened, it may easily determine itself to any other Subject, and so spoil your Undertaking.

Since at this stage we already work with highly purified substances, we must take care not to spoil the work with impurities. On the other hand, the fear of foreign Sulfur seems somewhat exaggerated, because the resinous matter also contains foreign Sulfur. The imbibition can also be done in a glass flask, which is then closed with a glass stopper.

Occasionally the flask is opened to allow for fresh air, then closed again. In this way I have obtained very workable results, but the flask must be quite large and contain much air. The danger of contamination is also greatly reduced by working in a closed oven (incubator).

XI

If in three, or four Weeks time at farthest, your fixt Vegetable Salt does not manifest its full Saturation, it will certainly be in vain for you to go on any further with it: for you may assure yourself, that you either err in the Notion of the Salt or of the real sulphureous Medium, or in the Management of the Imbibitions.

XII

When your Imbibitions are fully performed, your Salt will then be in a convenient readiness to receive its own Spirit, by which it is made volatil, spiritual, transparent, and wonderfully penetrating, entring on a sudden into the Pores and Particles of every Vegetable, and separating in a moment their true Essence or Elements.

If everything has gone well, we can now pour on our Mercury, that is, our rectified ethyl alcohol.

XIII

Altho the Salt is fully prepared for the Reception of its own Spirit, yet unless you well observe the right Proportion of them (which is, that the volatil always predominate over the fixt) you will never be able to make any perfect Union between these two Subjects, contrary in Quality, though not in Nature.

The mixture must be well covered by the alcohol. Even with a proportion of 6:1 or even 8:1, I have achieved good results. It is decisive for the whole work that we should have a sufficiently large quantity of proper essential oil. Like the anonymous Mercury in the plant world, alcohol is at any time easily available from outside sources.

XIV

Before you begin your Distillations and Cohobations, after the Addition of the Vegetable Spirit to its own Salt, a Putrefaction of eight to ten days is to precede, during which time, the sulphureous Spirit, strengthened by the bituminous Matter, and finding its Salt fit for Conjunction with it, has the power to enter into its Pores, to facilitate its Volatilization, and Union.

In the course of this putrefaction, which is nothing but a further digestion, a change in color occurs and the fine Salt appears like slime. The strengthened Sulfur and the Mercury now act upon the Salt and begin to make part of it volatile. After this, we begin with the distillations.

XV

If after six or seven Distillations and Cohobations of the distilled upon the Remainder, you do not find your Spirit to be extremely sharp, and the Remainder in the bottom altogether insipid, it will be an evident Sign, that you fail in the true knowledge of the Vegetable Spirit, which, being exceeding volatil, has in its Nature power to volatilize its own Body, and unite itself inseparably with it, finding it capable of its Reception.

The fractionating flask is best heated in the water bath. Between the separate distillations, or cohobations—since the distillate is always poured back—additional digestions are occasionally useful, but they are not prescribed. After six or seven distillations, or cohobations, the distillate has a peculiar, very penetrating odor and a sharp corrosive taste.

XVI

It is to be observed, that in the Progress of your Distillations the sulphureous Medium does not in the least ascend: for as it is a real Medium, concurring to unite the Body with the Spirit, before the Spiritualization of the Body, and without the Concurrence of which no perfect Union of these two Subjects is to be expected; so on the contrary in the Progress of the Work its Concurrence would be highly disadvantageous to them both, and totally subvert your Operation.

To avoid this, we make our distillations in the water bath. The resinous matter must not be distilled over or burn. It has accomplished its function as an intensifier of the Sulfur, and we no longer need the rest. Too-high temperatures would also rather result in a fixation of the volatile parts of the fixed Salt instead of its volatilization. We would then end with a solid substance instead of a Circulatum. Careful and slow distillations are therefore necessary, just as they are in all attempts at volatilizing alkaline Salts. It is here where the practicing alchemist can make many mistakes. Much patience and experience are needed for these distillations.

Otherwise what may happen is what Urbigerus describes in the following aphorism:

XVII

The ascending of the sulphureous Medium, when the Spirit begins to carry over its own Body, to unite itself inseparably, with it, evidently and certainly signifies, that you do not regulate your Fire, as you should, and that, instead of giving a gentle vaporous Heat to facilitate the Union, you give a violent one to destroy it.

XVIII

When your Salt is brought to its perfect Spiritualization, and real Union with its own Volatile Spirit, then you will have in your power your Circulatum Minus, or Vegetable Elixir, and Menstruum, with which you will be able to perform wonders in the Vegetable Kingdom, separating in a moment not only their Principles or Elements, but also at one and the same Operation the Pure from the Impure.

If all works have been correctly carried out, the alchemist has now prepared the Circulatum Minus according to the third way.

From all that has been said, the first way is now also easily understandable, as everything has simply to be prepared from the same plant species from which the resinous matter comes; for instance, you could make a Circulatum Minus from the North American *Abies balsamea*. The resinous matter can be extracted from small branches by steam distillation. In this way natural turpentines are obtained. The remaining operations are then carried out according to the methods already described.

In the following aphorisms Urbigerus now informs us about everything the Circulatum Minus, thus prepared, can do.

XIX

If into this your Vegetable Elixir you put any green Vegetable, shred in pieces, it will in less than half a quarter of an hour without any external Heat putrify, and precipitate itself into the bottom quite dead, (which is nothing but the cursed Excremental Earth) and on the top will swim a yellow Oil, containing the Salt and Sulphur, and the Elixir will be of the Color of the Plant, comprehending its Vegetable Spirit; which if it does not, 'tis a sign, that your Operations have not been Philosophical.

After immersing a finely cut green, that is, fresh, plant—for instance, peppermint or rosemary leaves—there will at first, after shaking, occur a strong turbidity. This turbidity is a sign of the emulsion now obtained. If we allow it to stand for some time, the tiny droplets of oil will rise to the surface, where they form a yellowish layer of oil. This oil contains the Salt and the Sulfur of the fresh plant or plants immersed in the Circulatum. In my experience, the color of the oil varies according to the plants used. Some produce a more yellowish oil, others a shining emerald one. With other plants the oil is orange or reddish.

Depending on the specific weight of the Circulatum, also of the plants that we separate, the oil also occasionally settles at the bottom instead of floating on the surface. If we incline the vessel, the pearls of oil then appear.

XX

Only one drop of this yellowish Oil, given in Distempers according to the Virtue and Quality, attributed to the Plant, every Morning and Evening in a Glass of Wine, or any other convenient Vehicle, will infallibly and insensibly cure those Distempers, and corroborate the vital Spirits, if constantly taken to purify the Blood in sickly and infectuous Times.

I would here like to warn the reader, however, not simply to trust all information. In the alchemistic literature fantastic effects are often claimed, which are by no means always proven. Only experience, in collaboration with qualified physicians and naturopaths, can prove the value of a preparation. The value, or the worthlessness, of a spagyric preparation must be honestly tested if alchemy is to be taken seriously, and in this connection the laws in force in each country must be considered.

XXI

If you put Coral into this Menstruum, you will see an admirable Experiment: for although its Pores are compacter, than in any other Vegetable; yet it will on a sudden transmit its internal Spirit into the Menstruum, and sending its Soul and Body, like a blood-red Oil to the Top, will at last fall to the Bottom like a greyish Excrement.

XXII

If Myrrh, Aloe, and Saffron, of each an equal Quantity, are put into this Menstruum, the truest Elixir Proprietatis (as Paracelsus terms it) which is a most excellent Cordial, and almost of as great Efficacy and Virtue, as the Universal Elixir itself, and curing all curable Distempers, will presently swim on the Top, and its Caput Mortuum will separate itself into the Bottom.

XXIII

This Vegetable Menstruum dissolves not only all sorts of Gums, or any other kind of Substance in the Vegetable Kingdom, but also all sorts of Oils and Balsams, coming out of Trees, separating their true Essence, by which you may perform wonderful things both upon living Bodies, and dead ones, the last of which it preserves forever without opening or any further Preparation of them.

XXIV

Though this Menstruum is only specificated upon Vegetables, it will nevertheless in a moment draw the Tincture out of Metals and Minerals; but it will not separate all their Principles, not being the appropriate Menstruum for such Operations; and though such Sulphurs are highly balsamic for the Lungs and Spleen, yet since our Elixir Proprietatis far exceeds those praeter natural Preparations, we only give this as a curious Chymical Experiment.

Aphorisms XXI–XXIV give us further pointers for the use of the Circulatum. Aphorism XXII is especially important in connection with the previous chapter on the plant magistery of Paracelsus. An immersion of equal quantities of myrrh, aloe, and saffron results in the famous Elixir Proprietatis of Paracelsus. If we use the Circulatum Minus of Urbigerus, a simple immersion is enough to bring about the separation, and we need then no longer rotate a whole month as with the "simple" Paracelsian magisteries. The Circulatum Minus of Urbigerus is really a Circulatum "of high degree," as the ancients would say. It also immediately dissolves various lacs, oils, and balsams. Be careful: with a minute amount I instantly ruined the finish of my desk!

In addition, the Circulatum extracts the tincture from certain metals. These tinctures, however, do not represent true separations.

There is a great difference between the simple extraction of a tincture and a genuine separation of the Philosophical Principles. To separate metals higher Circulata are required, namely the high Alkahests, whose preparation does not concern us here.

Aphorism XXV now describes how we can regain our Circulatum after a separation.

XXV

Since this Vegetable Menstruum is eternal, you must observe, that you lose nothing of its Quantity or Quality in separating it from the Oil, and Spirit of the Vegetable, which is done by a gentle Distillation in Balneo vaporoso, the Vessel being very well luted and dried before. The Menstruum, coming over with the Flegm of the Vegetable, from which it is by a Distillation in Balneo to be separated for further uses, leaves the Oil at the Bottom, united with its own Spirit, which will easily go over in any common Heat, not leaving anything behind it: which is a Mark of its Spiritualization, Purification, and Regeneration, that it has received from the Menstruum.

With this we will end this chapter on the Circulatum Minus.

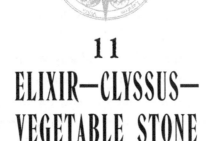

11
ELIXIR–CLYSSUS–
VEGETABLE STONE

I n chapter 5 we dealt with the *Solve* of the alchemistic work and learned how to separate a plant into its Essentials or Philosophical Principles. We kept these Essentials for a later combination. The *Coagula* is the reunion of the previously separated Principles. In the classical spagyrico-medicinal literature, the terms *Elixir, Clyssus,* and *Lapis Vegetabilis* (Vegetable or Plant Stone) often turn up. We shall now deal with them.

In modern pharmacology the term *elixir* means a sweetened, aromatic solution, mostly on the basis of a water-alcohol mixture, which has a specific effect on the organism. The significance of the term *elixir* deteriorated in the course of time by designating as elixirs even nonmedical solutions that were only used as vehicles for flavors or other substances.[50] In the spagyric tradition, an Elixir is a pharmaceutical product prepared from several different species of plants. What is decisive is the formula for the composition in quantity and kind as well as the method of preparation. The greatest importance is attached to the widest possible utilization of the species. It is not a question of fragmented products such as mixtures of essential oils, tinctures poured together, and the like.

The classical Elixirs always contain the Salts that are extracted through incineration and calcination of the plant residue. In the later

literature Elixir recipes also turn up that do not always contain the calcined Salts. Often in later times certain herb and spice teas were also
called Elixirs. In the strictly spagyric sense, however, only those products
are Elixirs that have been prepared in the philosophical manner, that
is, spagyrically, from several plants, and it is assumed that they contain
the calcined Salts. Depending on their composition, Elixirs have specific effects on the organism: some stimulate the circulation, others help
digestion or sleep, others again have a cathartic effect, and so forth. In
former times the so-called Life Elixirs or cordials were popular. They
were general tonic Elixirs.

The Integral Herbal Elixirs of Australerba in Australia are genuine
spagyric Elixirs in the sense just discussed. Elixirs are taken either with
a spoon or thinned with water or wine. The popular Australerba Elixirs
are thinned in hot water and taken as herb teas. The Australerba Elixirs also contain some citrus pectin, which tones the digestive tract up
and helps metabolize toxic food residues, balance excessive gastric acidity, and lower cholesterol levels. Pectins strengthen the resistance of the
digestive organs.[51]

Since pectin is hard to dissolve in cold liquids, however, Australerba
also offers Elixirs without pectins. They are preferably taken in sweet
wines, which are thus transformed into pleasant herb wines.

As an example from the classical literature, here now follows the
recipe for a Life Elixir (tonic) that Andreas Libavius has given us.[52]

Macerate for one month in 2 or 3 pounds of good Greek wine [or,
more quickly, one can boil for half a day in a diploma]: Of each of the
following 3 drams [c. 11.6 grams] of wood of aloe, sweet-smelling
costus, white and yellow sandalwood; of each 2 drams [c. 7.8 g] of
angelica root, lovage, burnet saxifrage, masterwort, canine thistle,
and spicknel; half an ounce each [c. 15.55 g] of valerian, white
dittany, peony, oak mistletoe, bloodwort, and lemon, orange, and
lime peels; 5 drams each [c. 19.4 g] of lemon, avens seeds, laurels,
juniper berries, and peony seeds; and 6 drams [c. 23.3 g] of Alpine
colt's foot; everything to be pulverized.

Now take 5 ounces [c. 155.5 g] of mace, nutmeg, long pepper, zedoary, and cloves; 2 drams each [c. 7.8 g] of seeds of cardamom, marjoram, and basil; 1½ drams [5.8 g] of saffron; half a handful each of flowers of sage, rosemary, hedge-nettle [also known as woundwort, stachys], bugloss [Anchusa], and borage; and one handful each of marjoram, basil, pennyroyal, mint, and sage.

First, after cutting and chopping them up, make an infusion of the aromatic herbs and the seeds in a sufficient quantity of water, and let it stand for ten days in moderate digestion. After separation through a percolator and by pressing, the rest is to be macerated in the liquid, chopped up in the same way, for five days.

Now the first infusion is also filtered and pressed and then united with the second. In the extracts poured together, dissolve 1 ounce [c. 31.1 g] of mithridate [dogtooth violet], half an ounce each [c. 15.55 g] of treacle and *Aurea Alexandrina,* and 6 drams each [c. 23.2 g] of *Gallia muschata,* and a preparation of pokeberries. After three days of maceration, one should distill. The collected residue is now burnt to ash by a reverberating fire, and the alkali (the salts) are extracted with betony water. Mix this with the distillate and add 2 pounds [c. 746.5 g] of sugar dissolved in the fourfold quantity of rosewater, and one scruple [c. 1.3 g] of distillated oil of cloves, cinnamon, nutmeg, and lemon peel.

In a specially preserved part, hang also half a scruple each [c. 0.64 g] of golden amber and musk. Thus the Elixir is to be made.

Although not all Elixirs are as complicated to compound and prepare, their preparation nevertheless always requires several fairly long operations. We are dealing with products in which several kinds of extracts are combined together. Often several extracts are made one after another. The plant residue is then dried, incinerated, and calcined; the salts are extracted and added to the Elixir. Frequently, still further additions follow, such as spices, distilled oils, pectins, resins, and so on, including mineral preparations for some Elixirs.

The separate times of maceration or digestion vary with the plants, as does the water-alcohol proportion. With plants with a high content of essential oils, the alcohol content of the solvent is higher. Certain aromatic substances are also extracted under higher temperatures in the reflux system. Because of the instability of alkaloids, it is best to extract alkaloid-containing plants cold or with only moderate heat.

The preparation of Elixirs requires a thorough knowledge and experience, since an exchange of powers and substances takes place among the species.

Anyone who wants good recipes should hunt for them by studying old texts and manuscripts. Many of the Elixirs in them were prepared with simple technical aids.

If the Elixirs are mixtures of extracts of various species of plants, the Clyssus (also written *Clissus*) is a preparation of recombined extracts of only one plant. In his *Magiae naturalis libri viginti*, Johannes Baptista Porta says, "The Clyssus is the extraction of the subtlety of all parts of the plant, which flows together into a common being."[53]

A Clyssus is always prepared from the whole plant. The plant, together with everything belonging to it, that is, root, blossoms, stem, leaves, fruits, seed, and so on, is first separated in the classical manner, that is, separated into the three Essentials, Mercury, Sulfur (volatile and fixed), and Salt, after which the Essentials are recombined. In so doing, either the fixed Sulfur is used as resinous matter, or it is incinerated and calcined, and the salts are extracted. These are then added to the Clyssus.

The reunion of Sulfur, Salt, and Mercury hardly gives trouble, as everything can simply be recombined. The salts are imbibed with Mercury, to which is added the volatile Sulfur, or the Sulfur is first poured on the salts, and then Mercury is added. The imbibition is to be done gradually until the salt no longer absorbs anything. In this state the Clyssus thus prepared can be melted and poured into a form to cool. It is a kind of simple Plant Stone that contains, in a concentrated form, certain curative powers of the plants from which it derives. Due to the strong concentration of the salts, it has quite a diuretic and purging effect, and it also improves digestion. If we wish to make a more liquid Clyssus, it must contain one part of water to dissolve the salts. In this case, it is best to use water extracted from the relevant plant by distillation, or else residual water from our Mercury rectification, or distilled water. We pour on the salt only as much water as is needed to dissolve it. Then we add the volatile Sulfur and the Mercury. Without Mercury, the volatile Sulfur would float on the water. Only Mercury can combine the oily with the watery parts.

A Clyssus can be highly concentrated but also rather thinned, according to the individual practice of the spagyrist. In his *Chymischer Handleiter,* Le Febure advises the following proportions: one part Salt, two parts Sulfur, and three parts Mercury. These quantities result in a more solid Clyssus.

Among the classical recipes we also find pointers on how to combine the Essentials by means of a simultaneous distilling apparatus. To this end, we put the three Essentials into three different flasks, which then go under one alembic for distilling and are distilled through a common condenser. Leonhardt Thurneysser zum Thurn describes the process in his *Historia.*[54] He refers to a Clyssus made of olysatrum (Macedonian parsley). The difficult original text is here summarized in modern English on account of its importance:

Paracelsus calls Clyssus not only the medicament described in the following lines but also that other power which originally stems from one thing alone [a single species], after this species has separated into different parts and finally recombines into one thing.

If seed is put into the soil, the root system develops first, then the plant grows, which then forms the flower, followed by the fruit, and finally the seed.

Each of these individually formed morphological parts has its special properties. That is why out of each its proper power is extracted. The relevant individual powers are then combined into a single power.

Such a preparation can be an oil, for instance, or an Arcanum [a secret medicine, prepared in a higher way], furthermore a juice, a powder, a salt, etc., which is then called Clyssus.

An estate which a father bequeaths to his many children and which then reverts to one child alone because of the death of the brothers and sisters, can also be called a Clyssus.

We will here, however, understand the term in the above-described sense. The preparation of a Clyssus is done as follows:

From the three parts (roots, stem with leaves, and flowers, fruit, and seed)—provided that at the right time the roots of the plants were dug up, the plants harvested, and the seeds gathered, hence from the perfectly full-grown roots, plants, flowers, fruits, and seeds—the power and subtlety of each are separately extracted either through distillation, calcination, putrefaction, or other methods, corresponding in each case to the nature of the species used.

Since every plant has its specific shape and property, the relevant correct extraction process must be applied in each case, corresponding with the teaching and explanation of the properties of things accessible to intelligent people.

After the subtle powers have been separated one by one, first as an oil, second as a salt, third as a liquid (or whatever we may wish to call them) from the individual plant parts of the species, they are recombined in the following manner into a single spiritual substance and an inseparable being:

We put the previously extracted subtleties into three equally large flasks, the lower part of which is coated with loam as protection from fire (see B, C, and D of the diagram), that is, the salt into flask B, the oil into flask C, and the liquid into flask D. Now we attach a wide-necked alembic, which covers the three openings of the flask simultaneously and equally well, and we seal well with Lutum [an adhesive paste made of clay]. If the three flasks are now simultaneously heated, the subtlety rises upward from each, at the same time becoming volatile with the other two and ascending into the alembic.

The soul powers at first mingle as steam, which then precipitates as moisture (as "moist fruit"). The moisture is brought out through the beak [of the alembic] and is born in this way. The receiver E absorbs what is born as would a nurse. This Clyssus is a very useful Arcanum.

The drawing at the beginning of the original text represents a simultaneous distilling apparatus. With this kind of preparation, problems arise from the fact that the Essentials have different high boiling points; they do not rise at the same temperature.

When using this kind of apparatus, the salts are often dissolved in water before the distillation. Then, during the distillation, they are brought over the alembic partly volatilized. To achieve this, cohobations are frequently required. The Clyssus prepared in this way is in a thin liquid state.

Now follows another recipe from the *Chymischer Handleiter* of Le Febure.[55] It refers to a Clyssus of angelica; strictly speaking, Le Febure describes a Clyssus made with the roots of angelica:

The rest is preserved so that, if one wishes to reunite or combine in one body all volatile as well as all fixed parts of the angelica root in order to make a Clyssus of them (which, like a summary, comprises in itself all the virtues of the Mirti, all the parts of which have separated and purified), one can unite the rectified spirit and the heavenly oil by means of the fixed Salt, for without it, the two above-mentioned could never be brought together into one body, because they have different natures and one is always floating on top of the other. But when the subtle and rectified spirit is united with its own Sal alkali, the oil can be mixed with it inseparably, from which a wonderful substance arises. As far as the Clyssus is concerned, however, it does not require so much effort. Only one part of the fixed purified Salt is to be put together with two parts of the distilled oil and three parts of the subtle spirit, and these are to be digested in a circulating vessel in B.V., until everything is quite exactly combined, which usually takes place in a philosophical

month, which has 40 days. This Refuedium, if it is prepared as indicated, can rightly be administered instead of the spirit-oil, extract,
and Salt, because it contains the powers of these four things. The
dose varies between six grains and one scruple in all diseases when
otherwise the angelica root from which it is prepared is used.

Here we recognize a somewhat different conception, the making of
a Clyssus from the root instead of the whole plant.

On the other hand, there are Clyssus recipes that prescribe the
complete utilization of all plant parts, even if they are only available in
different seasons. This is proven by the following recipe for a juniper
Clyssus by Andreas Libavius.[56]

One is to be distilled from the green berries, a second from the
black ones, a third from the bark, a fourth from the wood and the
root. From the shoots the viscus (thick juice) is to be prepared;
from the wood and the bark, the oil from one, the resin from the
other; from the residue, the salt (through incinerating, calcining,
leaching, and evaporating); from the whole plant, the alkali.[57] The
four waters are to be poured together and the salts dissolved in
them. Then the viscus and the resin are to be distilled into a balm.
The balm mixed with the oil is to be brought into the waters and
united with them through shaking and digesting, or at least it is to
be given together with the oil when administered. The substances
can also be turned into a form of electuary [confection] by forming the coarser ones into a paste which is to be imbibed by and by
with the waters.

Technically seen, this Clyssus is an emulsion, since no Mercury is added
in the form of alcohol that combines the oils with the waters. On the
other hand, an attempt is here made to extract the maximum from the
juniper plant.

A special technique is proposed by Porta in his *Magiae naturalis
libri viginti*. Should the Clyssus require the simultaneous distillation of

resinous substances, for instance of the fixed Sulfur, he proposes the apparatus shown in figure 47.

The resins are put at the bottom of the flask, the waters are above them in a cup. As the heat is stronger under the resinous matter, the balsam of the resin is driven over faster, so that it can unite with the watery vapors during distillation, as Porta expresses it, "in the manner of spirits."[58]

Let us now turn to the preparation of a solid Vegetable Stone, also called Plant Stone. We have just seen that there are different views about the concept of Clyssus. It is similar with the Stones.

We have already made the acquaintance of the liquid Plant Stone in connection with the Circulatum Minus. It has the ability to separate.

Although in alchemical circles it is often said that the fixed Plant Stone can also separate, I am skeptical about this assertion, as I do not find it confirmed in the majority of the texts on this subject or in practice. The tiny "small membrane" that appears on top when a fixed Plant Stone is brought into maceration does not represent a real separation, in my view. Anyone who has experienced a genuine separation with the Circulatum will never confuse it with the effect of the Plant Stone on fresh plants in water. For a separation the liquid Plant Stone is used, the Circulatum. The medicinal value of the Plant Stone, however, is always greatly stressed in the relevant works. Conversely, the Circulatum Minus

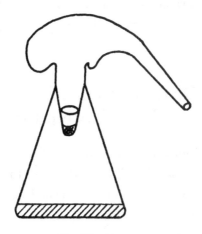

Fig. 47

itself is not a medicine; it serves only to separate the oils and magisteries that then have great medicinal value.

In alchemy, there are Stones and Stones. Texts and practice, however, make it plain that a genuine Lapis Vegetabilis, in the true sense of the word, is more than a Clyssus, insofar as in the last part of its preparation it must always go through the slow process of fixation in the fixing glass. Later, the glass is broken and the Stone taken out, or it is cast while still hot. Fixation takes place in a hermetically sealed glass through prolonged heating in a hot-air furnace, the Athanor. This applies to Stones from fresh plants, dry plants, honey, and also from wine.

Nonfixed compounds of Salts, Sulfur, and Mercury are stonelike compounds and certainly true spagyric preparations, but they are not Plant Stones in the higher and real sense.

Let us now consider some directions for the preparation of Plant Stones.

In the year 1659, the *Opus Vegetabile* of Johannes Isaac Hollandus was published in Amsterdam.[59] This text will now serve as the basis for three works.

The first concerns the preparation of the Plant Stone from dry herbs, the second its preparation from fresh herbs, the third its preparation from honey. In Hollandus's work, the Plant Stone is also designated as Quinta Essentia.

First, the unabridged original text is given in translation, followed each time by a brief summary of the necessary processes in modern language.

The *Opus Vegetabile* of M. Johannes Isaac Hollandus

Now my child should further know that I have said in the previous chapter that one should kill the herbs and let them die, and make a powder or ash of them. This is to be understood as follows: one should draw off the impure wateriness or let it dry of itself, which is best, or else draw it off in Balneo Mariae, because the bad moisture is what hinders the spirit most and keeps it imprisoned so that it cannot prove in man or in metals the power that is in ☿. The miserable simpletons work with the moisture, and if it should happen by chance that something good were done or discovered by them, the evil moisture would take from them what they were looking for. They set the herbs to putrefy, distill them afterward, and operate with the putrefied distillate. They take much trouble, but at the end everything the poor wretches have done is lost. Thus the Art seems impossible to them, and they begin to despise and slander it. Why have I said this? So that you should or might know where their mistake arises and what they are lacking. You might well believe that they separate the four Elements and wonder what the reason is that the spirits do not exercise their power. That, however, is because of the evil wateriness with which the herbs have been putrefied and with which they have worked. This is the reason and explanation; therefore guard against the evil wateriness. An accident known beforehand is more easily dealt with and prevented, and that is why I have told you about it.

Furthermore, when you now have distilled the evil moisture and the herbs are dry, distill the spirit per descensum, as I will teach you later, and calcine the Corpus till it is as white as snow. Now you have two natures, namely, body and spirit, and you can dissolve the spirit in very good Aqua Vitae, or in good distilled wine vinegar that is pure, and that is the liquid with which you should work. Dissolve also the Corpus in the same way as I have just taught regarding the spirit. Thus coagulated, you have two substances with which to work separately. But you still have no perfectly glorified Corpus, since the spirit is not yet united with the body and they are not yet married and combined. That is also why they do not yet have their perfect power, although they are clean and pure; and although they had been ash and water and have now again come alive, they still differ in as much as each is by itself. Nevertheless, each has a special power that it bestows, each in its own vehicle.

To better understand what I have said, you should know that there are two different kinds of diseases in man, and likewise in ☿ . In man is a disease called spiritual sickness, and still another disease called accidental sickness. However, I do not mean troubles of the soul when I speak of spiritual diseases, but I am of the opinion that men may well have different dispositions in their bodies. What I call spiritual sicknesses, however, are those that come upon man accidentally or by chance, such as are due to anger, fantasies, regrets, or grief, or to unexpected misfortunes, or losses, or too much studying, or too much stress on the senses, or anxiety, or afflictions of the senses, or fear and fright which befall men or are caused them, and too many other things that would take too long to describe here, all spiritual diseases from which severe sicknesses can result for man, that is, bad fevers, bad inflammatory diseases, and others too many to enumerate here. All those infirmities must be treated with the spirit of plants, provided they have been prepared by themselves, meaning that the spirit will purge them.

In addition, there are still other diseases in man which are called accidental, and these spring from too much eating and drinking, or from ingesting bad food and drink, or from overindulgence in eating and drinking after suffering great hunger and thirst. This results in bad diseases, abcesses, bad water-galls on the liver and spleen. The lungs are damaged through harmful cold and heat. In addition, the kidneys are injured through excessive feeding and too much incontinence, by which the blood of the loins is lost. These and similar diseases, of which there is a great number, are called accidental sicknesses, and they are cured with the body of the herbs, provided they are prepared in this way, and that is the plant body's power and effect. But when body and spirit are united, they have such a wonderful effect that no pen can describe how much power and virtue they have, and there is no master in the world who could completely fathom the power and capability that the Lord God has conferred upon them. Thus, the spirit of all plants, trees, and species is so noble that all the doctors in the world could not comprehend the "ancientness" of a single Spirit, even if it belonged to the very meanest little herb that God has created in the world. How could they know the powers of all plants, trees, and species, since every species has a particular nature and spirit? One spirit is always nobler than another.

I am well aware, however, that among all insensitive spirits none is as noble and efficacious as the excellent spirit of the noble vine, because God Almighty has provided from the beginning of time that the noble grape should grow on it, later to be changed into God's blood and body. Consequently, the wise know well that the spirit of wine surpasses all other spirits. This is the reason why the philosophers of old have found in no plants, trees, or species greater powers than in the spirit extracted from wine. That is why I may well state that the noble spirit of the vine is the noblest and best of all things. Accordingly, some spirits are nobler than others, but no one can measure or find their extreme power except God alone. The fattest plants, however, which carry seed, are best for making Salarmeniac [*sal ammoniacus,* or ammonia]. After these, the best are the hottest herbs, from which the most powerful and strongest Salarmeniac is made.

If now you wish to prepare a medicine that is to act upon metals and Mercury, you must take some hot and healthy plants or roots that neither human beings nor animals can use, and make Salmiac and an Elixir of them, as I will teach you later. But if you wish to make a medicine or Elixir for human beings, take nice, good plants that are helpful to people and which they can use. Make a medicine or Elixir of them with which you can operate inside man. Then you will achieve wonderful cures in man, so that the whole world will be surprised at you and everybody will wish to see you. Enough of this, but do understand me rightly as to what matter I have indicated to you by all possible means.

My child should also be aware that I have said and taught in the previous chapters how to recognize the nature of plants and how to separate their spirits from their bodies, and what is to be done with them. I will now explain and teach this better. Know that there is still another spirit of Salarmeniac, that is, one extracted from saline things, which is also Salarmeniac, because the spirits of all insensitive things are called Salarmeniac when they are separated from their bodies, so that the spirit of all salts is called Salarmeniac. But it is not the Salmiac that the Philosophi mean, the Salarmeniac extracted from plants, which contains the four Elements. That is the Salmiac which the Philosophi mean, and from the Salmiac they make Elixiria, but one cannot make Elixirs from the other kind. That is the philosophers' soap and washing water with which they clean the Corpora. With it they dry the evil moisture of the Elements, with it they also dissolve the Corpora, and with it they conjoin the things that are contrary or antagonistic to each other. It is a flying spirit, one that comes and goes, and if it were not present, the Elixir would not succeed. In this Salmiac there are many hidden things that cannot all be described, because wonderful things can be accomplished with it if it has previously been fixed. But that is not necessary for this work. However, everything the Salmiac from the salts achieves is also done by the Salmiac from the plants. And from the Salmiac extracted from the plants an Elixir can be made without the addition of other species—which cannot be done with the Salarmeniac from the salts. But that Salarmeniac can well be prepared with other species, so that with it the Mercury can be dissolved in water, likewise all other metals and all things, provided one proceeds with them as I have taught elsewhere. For now, enough of it.

Now I will teach my child further and describe the powers and virtues that plants have when the Elements have been purified, cleansed, calcined, distilled, and afterward recombined and made fixed, and a glorified Corpus has resulted from all this. Neither I myself nor all the doctors in the world can sufficiently understand the powers and nature that I have seen in them and tested, and of which the journeymen with whom I worked and other masters have told me. For no one but God can understand them when they have thus been prepared and turned into a perfect Corpus; no one can know it but God alone. He knows, and no one else.

In addition, you should know that there are many errors among those who work in this Art, which errors I have previously touched upon when I spoke of the evil wateriness that plants contain, with which they work and putrefy. Afterward, when they have distilled that wateriness off the plants, they call it the Element Water, but in the end they cannot achieve any perfection with it, of which I shall write more later. Here, however, I will teach how to separate the Elements. You should know that there are many kinds of separations, since there have been many artists who wished to learn the way of separating, because of which the Elements can then be separated in many different ways, but one separation is better than another, though both are good. We also find many simpletons among scholars and the illiterate who would also dare to undertake these works. They begin to work in the laboratory and imagine that they also have an understanding of the art of separation of the four Elements. Then they say that they have separated the four Elements one from another, each separately. And then they imagine that they have performed great wonders. They say, "We have made the Quinta Essentia." True, with it they drive away many diseases in man, because it has in itself much power and good virtue; that is certain, more than they themselves know. But that the miserable fools imagine that they have made the Quinta Essentia and separated the Elements one from the other, that is nothing but sheer deception. They may well have a great medicine, moreso than they realize. But that they pretend and say, "We have the Quinta Essentia," is far from true. You poor simpletons, you have no Quinta Essentia. Quinta Essentia is quite another thing than you believe. It is a glorified Corpus that has been brought to perfection and is fixed and lasts eternally. Whoever has that can say he has the Quinta Essentia. Such a person has an earthly treasure that is better than a kingdom, and it is a gift of God which He bestows especially upon His friends. Happy is the person who has attained it and knows how to use it well for the salvation of his soul and the benefit of the poor. He will fare well in this world and in the other. Instead, those who use these gifts of God differently shall have their troubles in this world and afterward suffer infinite torture in the eternal hellfire. Therefore, take care that you use this Art to the honor of God and the salvation of your soul. For I swear by the living God Who has created heaven and earth that, if you use this gift differently, you shall not live long and shall be tortured here in this world with temporal and afterward with eternal pain. Therefore, watch out what you are doing. It would be better for you never to have been born than to have the Art and misuse it. Therefore, you yourself must take great care. Enough said to those who understand.

Summary of the Processes

First, extract the "evil" wateriness from the plants, which is best done by drying them normally in a place sheltered from the sun, otherwise in a flask heated in a water bath.

When the plants are dry, the "spirit" is drawn off by a dry distillation (Descensum). Heat for twelve hours, draw the steam over, slowly increase the heat, then for twenty hours increase the heat even more, until finally the barrel (container) is red hot; then the red oil will also go over. In my experience, the Descensum can easily be performed in a strong flask with gas heating. The receiver now contains some distilled water, on top of which floats the evil-smelling oil. It is removed with a feather, as it will not become part of the work. The oil can be stored separately for other purposes. It is quite a dangerous substance and, in the view of Hollandus, can cause cancer. It is true that this oil, if rightly applied, has great curative powers.[60]

The distillate thus obtained is again distilled (in the water bath), then poured back on the residue (cohobation). The precipitating feces are filtered, and the distillate is once more distilled in the water bath. This process is repeated until everything is pure without feces.

The calcined residue (Earth) is now treated in like fashion. The Earth is calcined for three days, then ground with alcohol or distilled wine, again put in the water bath, the feces are filtered, again new alcohol is poured on, then again set in the water bath, then the liquid is filtered and poured back on that drawn off first. This process is repeated until everything is extracted from the fecibus. Now the alcohol is extracted through distillation, a white Corpus stays behind. By cohobating with alcohol, the Earth can be considerably fortified, especially by cohobating four times.

The purified Earth and the purified spirit are ground together, dissolved in water (according to other instructions, in the water of wine or alcohol), and digested for fifteen days in the water bath.

Now we distill again. Only water is allowed to go over; the Mercury combines. If spirits go over, we pour back (cohobate) after every distillation and again distill, until only a watery substance comes over.

We now put the residue into a flask and as much rectified water (alcohol or vinegar) as has been drawn off, until everything is dissolved. Gently we now let the water evaporate; we set everything into the athanor (laboratory furnace) for forty days, at summer temperature. Then the Stone can be cast.

Now follows Hollandus's text concerning the preparation of the Plant Stone from fresh plants.

Treatise

How to Make the Vegetable Stone or Quintam Essentiam from All Green Plants, Seeds, Roots, and the Like, from Which the Cloud-Water Goes Over First

Now you will learn another way of distilling plants, when the water goes over first, by which are understood all kinds of plants from which the cloud-water [ordinary water] rises over first [as steam]. For in connection with this operation and teaching everything that can be made from green plants and roots will be understood. After this, the teaching will concern all dry species, gums, woods, and everything that is dry, each taught separately.

Now my child should know that we wish to make the Vegetable Stone from green plants from which the cloud-water goes over first, and my child must know above everything at what time the plants are to be gathered and stored; when they have the greatest strength to prepare the Stone from them. Know then, my child, that plants have three ages. The first is when they are sprouting. Then they are like a newborn child without strength and power, who is moist and watery. Likewise with plants. The second age is like that of a man of twenty-five years. He is in the prime of life till his fortieth year. Likewise with plants as they are growing, until they begin to bloom and go to seed. Then they are in their flowering time until the seed is ripe. The third age is like that of a man from his fortieth to his eightieth year, when all his strength begins to disappear. Likewise with plants. When the seed is ripe, the plants begin to die and wither gradually until they are altogether gone.

Therefore my child should take the plants when they are full-grown and begin to go to seed or to ripen, because all plants begin to seed and are sometimes blooming at the same time. Accordingly, take the plants that you see have mostly gone to seed, although many of them are still blooming and do not yet bear seed. Pick them together with their leaves, flowers, roots, and seed, on a clear day, when the sun shines strongest. Clean them rapidly without washing them or adding any moisture; put them thus whole into a jar, packed as tightly as you can, up to the neck, add the alembic gently, and set it in the Balneum. Begin at once to distill so that you do not loose the wild spirits that fly away invisibly, about which I shall teach you in the treatise on the wine. The spirits are the greenness, the taste and the smell, and the life of the plants. That is why the philosopher Dantin says, "See to it that you carefully preserve your greenness, or you shall look in vain."

Now, my child, I have taught you at what time you should gather the plants. We shall now see from what plant we shall make this Vegetable Stone. To this end, we do not find a more common plant and one that is esteemed less than Chelidonia. I am telling you for certain, my child, that there are three plants that have preference over all others. They are Chelidonia, Solaria, and Lunaria. All are useful for the Art when they are prepared, and they congeal ☿ into true ☉ about which I will teach you in the work on the Mineral Stone. I am telling you, my child, that the noblest of all three is Chelidonia, because the other two die in winter, but Chelidonia always remains in its greenness and flowers. All other plants in the world wither and dry when it is warm in the summer, but this Chelidonia remains ever green, and even if it were lying under the snow through the winter, it would still not perish, neither in heat nor cold, dryness nor humidity. It is the very best and strongest of the three plants, but is not much esteemed because it is found in abundance. I am telling you, God has infused such an influence into this plant that no one can express it sufficiently. Therefore, my child, we will extract the other and second Vegetable Stone from it, to cure all men from their days of sickness and keep them healthy to the last hour of their lives; also to congeal ☿ into fine ☉. Accordingly, we will pick the plant when it is first flowering. Clean it and press it into three or four clean jars, as much as you can, without chopping it up. At once put an alembic on, set it in the Balneum to distill everything, draw all the water off until it is dry enough to be pulverized, then grind it on a stone with its water, so that one could paint with it, and put it into a big stone jar. When you have filled four or five jars with Chelidonia, put all the matter together into a stone jar. You must start with many plants in order to obtain much matter and much water. These plants, since they are not chopped up, take up much room.

But my child might ask: Why do you not chop up the plants? Know then that if the plants were crushed, part of the three spirits would fly away, namely, the greenness or color, and part of the air or taste, and part of the natural warmth, since the three spirits are so volatile that they do not permit any pounding or crushing.

You would therefore lose the major part of them, and afterward your work would be spoiled. You would only treat a dead Corpus, deprived of its soul and life, because the plant is mortified by crushing it. Try it: pound a green plant very small in a mortar. It will quickly lose its green color and natural moisture, since the whole house where the pounding is done is filled with the smell of the plant. The smell, however, no longer comes back after the nature of the plant has been broken and is mortified, so that it is, so to speak, alienated from the nature and influence of heaven, which cause its smell to grow. Also, heaven and the stars, which give or radiate their influence into it, no longer help it because it is broken, so that it no longer gets help from any source. Accordingly, immediately separate from it the three volatile spirits which are its Soul and Quinta Essentia. You understand, therefore, that plants cannot suffer any pounding or crushing, no more than a human being wants to be chopped to pieces, because the soul, which is his life, would at once escape from him. Consequently, my child, do not crush any green plant, but do as is taught above, so that you do not work with a dead body, which has been sufficiently proved before.

Now we go to our work. All that has been left over, you must pulverize on a stone. Put everything together into a big jar, place it into a lukewarm Balneum, pour its own water on it, stir it well with a wooden spoon, put a small ground glass on the mouth, let it stand thus for two days and two nights, stir it well every fourth or fifth hour, so that the water can draw out the Elements well. At the end of the two days, remove the can, set it aside, let it settle for three or four days, then pour the clear liquid from the fecibus into another jar, filter it, put the liquid into another jar—it is a golden water—plug it up well, and preserve it. Now again pour other water on the feces and stir well.

It would also be good if it were well dried before the water is poured on it, etc. Set it again in the Balneum for two days and two nights, stir it as before, cover it, etc. After this, let it cool, do as before, pour the water to the first, take once again some water and pour it on the feces. Do this until the feces no longer color the water; then you have the Air and the Fire out of the Earth, and the pouring has been sufficient. But should it happen that you have not enough water from the plants, you can take common water that has been twice or three times distilled per Balneum, and extract with it all Vegetable works, provided it is well distilled so that it does not leave any more feces. Then it is good for all green plants. With dry plants, however, one cannot extract or distill with common water, only, with distilled aceto. When the water has thus been distilled from the plants, take care of it, do your best, and extract the Elements with common water.

Now, my child, we will return to our work, to rectify our Air and Fire again together and to purify them of their fecibus. Pour all the colored water into a clean dish. Then take the white of 40 or 50 eggs, beat them quite thin like water, then beat them for half an hour together with the water, so that everything is well mixed. Now put the kettle over the fire, let it gently get warm and finally boil, but do not stir it at all. Then remove it from the fire. Have at hand a big white woolen Ypocras-bag. Pour all your water into it, let it percolate into a glass dish, and when it no longer drips, take distilled water and pour it upon the coagulated egg white. Let it sink through the feces in order to draw the Elements out of the fecibus. Do this as long as the feces color the water. Then you have extracted all the Elements. Dry the feces in a pan and keep them. They must be put back into the Earth in the flask to extract from them the combustible oil with the Salarmeniac, because there are many feces in the water of the egg whites. After this, take the liquid out of the bag, put it in the Balneum, stir it well, and let it stand for 24 hours in the warm Balneo, occasionally stirring it with a spoon, and cover the mouth again with some cut glass. Then take it out, let it settle for three or four days, then tip it gently to one side and pour it off gently per filtrum. See if you can find some feces at the bottom. If not, it is clarified enough; but if you find feces, it is not clear and must again be clarified as before.

My child should know the following regarding all things in the world: If one draws their water off dry per distillations, so that they turn to powder, and then crushes and percolates them, afterward pulverizes them on a stone, and if one again pours on them the water that had been drawn off from them, or other common distilled water, and one sets it in the Balneum, the water attracts to itself all Elemental Water, Air, and Fire. It turns red, and the redness lies in the innermost of the greenness that the plant has, and when it is congealed and dissolved with the water, it always precipitates its feces. If one repeats the operation frequently, it will finally clean and purify itself until no more feces precipitate. Yet this is a long way, and it takes less time with the white of eggs. But in regard to the green plants that have been dried in the sun and pulverized, even if you poured on them all the water in the world, it would not extract or color anything—they must be extracted with distilled vinegar. Further, the vinegar will not turn red but rather a bad yellow, since the plants have lost the greenness which had been their life, soul, and Quinta Essentia. The yellowness comes from the Elements that are still in it (the vinegar), but the three spirits are usually gone, and it is a dead corpse. It may still contain something of the Elements, so that it would like to do something, but it is not worth the trouble to work on it. Therefore, mark well what I am saying.

Now we shall recapitulate. If you find no more feces at the bottom of the jar, you must pour all the liquids together into a stone jar, set it in the Balneum, and distill off all the water, but not totally, so that you can pour the feces from the jar into a glass vessel, otherwise you will have to break the jar. After this, set the glass into a basin of sand, and set this basin on top of a basin of water. Into that, put the glass with the matter; let the water boil and the matter evaporate to dryness. Then take it out and break the glass, and your matter is clear, dry, and red; thus you have the Elemental Water, Fire, and Air. As to your three spirits, of which I have told you before, you have rectified and coagulated them to a Massa, but they are not fixed. Put them in your dry room until we need them.

In this way, my child, the Elemental Fire, the Elemental Water, and the Elemental Air, together with the three spirits, must all six be extracted from the Earth, without distilling, in the form of a Massa. They cannot be extracted from the Earth in any other way, since the three spirits, of which I have spoken before, rest in natural warmth and heat, that is, in taste, tincture, and smell. These three do not suffer any heat given by fire, for if one were to extract Water, Air, and Fire from the Earth through distilling, it would have to be done with the hot dryness from fire, ashes, or sand. If done in the Balneum, the Elemental Water, Air, and Fire will not rise, solely the cloud-water. If one wished to drive the Elemental Water, Air, and Fire over through distilling, it would have to be done by fire, while the three aforesaid Spirits cannot stand the heat given by fire. They would evanesce invisibly, and then you would lose their life, soul, and Quinta Essentia, and you would have instead a dead Corpus. Nevertheless, you would have the four Elements together, but they would be devoid of their Soul and their Quinta Essentia, which keep the four Elements together and connect them. For when these three Spirits are separated, the four Elements cannot stay together but must depart from each other and begin to decay and die, each Element returning to its nature, such as Air to Air, Fire to Fire, Water to Water, Earth to Earth, etc. Take, for instance, a man who has died and his natural warmth is gone. Soon the color that was in the blood, his natural smell and taste, all three are separated from man, which three are the soul that keeps the body together in one being. Understand well, my child, what it is when a child is conceived in its mother's womb by natural means. Within forty days a human being is formed; all members are perfectly arranged through the warmth of nature that the mother has in her blood, because the three spirits rest in the blood as in the natural warmth, smell, and taste. From the woman's blood the members are formed with the help of nature, as it has pleased God, and thus these three spirits rest in the woman's blood, and the child's members are formed with the aid of nature. Since these three spirits are in all the child's forms and members, when his parts are formed, that is, within 40 days, they are at first so tender and small as if they were threads, and he is like a little seed. Therefore, there cannot be much of these three spirits in him, and as slight as the little members are, God sends the soul into them, which comes from His supreme Will, springing from it in quite a miraculous manner, of which nothing will be said here because it does not belong to the matter under discussion. The soul has an eternal Essence, without beginning, in God; that is why it comes out of God, and the little members are not formed too small for the soul to come into being and at once operate in the body. For if the Soul did not enter it immediately, the three spirits would escape from it. That is why all three spirits must first be in the human being before the soul flows into it, and the three spirits keep the soul together in the body. As long as these three spirits are in the body, the soul also remains, and when the body becomes bigger, older, and stronger, these three spirits also gradually become bigger, older, and stronger. That is why they are called growing spirits. And as fast as these three spirits leave the Corpus, the soul must follow and vacate the body, because it has no place where it can rest. Try this with a man as soon as he is dead: cut, do what you want, you will not find any blood in him, or warmth, or smell, only a stench. Nevertheless the four Elements are in the corpse, namely, the Elemental Fire, Air, Water, and Earth, mixed with their stinking fecibus, but the Quinta Essentia is gone. That is, the three spirits: the natural warmth, the color, and the air. God has devised these three, and when these three spirits escape from the Elements, they do not stay together any longer. Each withdraws to where it came from; nothing remains but stinking feces. If one knew this, all works would proceed better, but they do not notice that no Spirit will stay in the body without a medium, to keep the spirit together with the body. They do not know that the media must be spirits that are quite volatile and are in the depth of matter. To the ignorant it is an unknown spirit. More of it will be explained in the Mineral Stone.

Understand also, my child, what these three spirits are, because if you do not know these three spirits and their nature, you will not succeed either in plant, animal, or mineral matters, but you will treat a dead Corpus. Therefore, according to the above-mentioned evidence, these three spirits can be drawn over with fire and air, so that they congeal together into a Massa, but in no way different from the one we have just taught. Do not look for any other media, or you will lose the three spirits invisibly and will then have a dead Corpus. Understand my words well—they are open words without any hidden meaning—so that you should not fall into error.

Now we shall recapitulate. Take all the feces that have remained in the jar and the white of the eggs with which you have clarified and which also contain feces. Put everything into a big earthenware retort, well sealed outside, as has been taught in the Work of the Wine, set it in a furnace in such a way that the fire and the flames can get at it on all sides. Attach to the retort a big stone jar almost full of distilled water and seal it quite tightly. First use a small fire, increased every three hours during 24 hours, then let it glow gradually, becoming stronger by and by, until the vessel is red-hot all around. Keep it standing thus for six hours. Within that time, the combustible oil will go over together with the Salarmeniac. Let it cool, then remove the jar and pour everything together into a big earthenware well-glazed cupel. Let it stand for three or four days, then the combustible oil will rise to the top. Take it off carefully, as cleanly as possible. Put the wet stuff that is in the cupel into a big stone can and preserve it until you are ready to rectify by coagulating and dissolving. Now take the combustible oil and put it into a small container, about which instructions have been given in the Work of the Wine. Pour boiling distilled water upon it, start clarifying as if you were making butter, just as has been taught in the Work of the Wine, where the combustible oil is purified of the Salarmeniac. It is all one operation. When the oil is pure, put it into a clean glass; use it for all sufferings that come from cold and liquid diseases, to clean lame limbs, and for paralysis. After this, take the water in which the combustible oil has been purified and the water from which the combustible oil has been taken off. Set everything together to coagulate in a Balneum, then let the feces sink, draw them off per filtrum, as has been taught in the Work of the Wine, to rectify it of the Salarmeniac, and when your Salarmeniac is well rectified and quite dry, white as snow, store that also in a dry room.

After this, take all the feces that have remained in the retort, also those left in the rectification, set them all together to reverberate, as has been taught in the Work of the Wine, until they become snow-white. Then rectify them again by pouring distilled water upon them, and let the water stand over them. After this, let the feces settle, then distill per filtrum and congeal again. Do this as has been taught in the Work of the Wine until your Earth is as white as snow. Then take the white Earth, dissolve it in your rectified water, put your Salmiac into the same water, distill the water dry to powder, then put it into the egg, calcine it in the secret furnace, and proceed in everything just as has been taught in the Work of the Wine. When you have calcined it in the manner taught in the said Work, etc., the Salarmeniac is ready to make the Stone. Now take your Fire and Air and your Elemental Water, as also your Earth, dissolve them together in Aqua rectificata, coagulate again, then put it in the egg, as is taught in the Work of the Wine, hang it in the secret furnace, and proceed as above. When everything is calcined, dissolve it in your Aqua rectificata, let the feces sink, draw it per filtrum, coagulate, and do as before until no more feces are left. Thereafter coagulate your Elemental Water, Fire, Air, and Earth once more; then you have your Massa rectificata of external and internal fecibus, in addition to your Salmiac, and they are now ready for you to make of them the Vegetable Stone.

Now take a large Receptacul, as is taught in the Work of the Wine. Put in it your Sal Armeniac, Elemental Water, Air, Fire, and Earth, plus their three spirits. Pour upon them some of your Aqua rectificata which has been drawn off from them, enough to dissolve well, but no more. Now set it into a crucible with sifted ashes, cover the glass with a small ground glass, not sealed but with a weight upon it. For 24 hours give if fire as warm as midsummer sunshine, then let it cool, pour it into the egg, and set it into a crucible with sifted ashes; let it evaporate with gentle heat until it is all quite dry, which you should test with a whetted knife put on the mouth of the neck of the egg. See if it is covered with vapor. If no moisture appears, it is dry; but to be more assured of it, let it stand in the heat for three or four days. Following this, seal it well with luto Herme-tis, and hang it in the secret furnace for 40 days, with heat like the summer sun or somewhat warmer.

After the 40 days, let it cool, remove the powder, and break the glass. Take the powder, put it into a crucible of Venetian glass, set it on burning coal, and the powder will melt like glass. Pour it into a small glass form that has previously been coated with oil. When it is cold, it is hard as stone, clear as crystal, red like a ruby, and trans-parent. This is the second Vegetable Stone which cures all diseases and infirmities in the world. If you take of it, in wine, every day, the equivalent in weight of a grain of wheat, you will see wonders after wonders in a few days.

Summary of the Processes

Especially suitable for the work are celandine, solaria, and lunaria. Whole, full-grown plants are cleaned but not washed. With these we fill a flask to the rim. We distill to dryness (draw off the moisture). Accord-ing to Hollandus, fresh herbs must not be ground, as it would lead to a loss of the spirits and the astrological influences.

Now the plants are pulverized. The triturated plants are then ground with the distilled water and are again put into the flask. More distilled water is added. We let everything stand for two days and two nights. Every four to five hours we stir with a wooden spoon. Now we let the feces settle for three to four days, then pour the water off on top and filter, the water has a golden color. We put it aside.

The residue in the flask is extracted in the same way with distilled water, until there is no more coloring.

The feces are now dried in a pan and then added to the Earth in order to extract from it the bad-smelling and combustible oil as well as the Salarmeniac.

The filtered liquid that has been passed through the wool bag is distilled to dryness in the water bath; the water is then poured back, and everything remains in the water bath for twenty-four hours. Now we filter and observe whether any feces are precipitating. If some feces appear, we clarify as before. If no feces fall out, we have done enough.

If the work is done in this way, the water draws all the Elemental Water, Elemental Air, and Elemental Fire out of the ground plant powder. This extract is red. The redness lies hidden in the greenness.

Purification can also be done by repeatedly distilling, dissolving, filtering, and renewed distilling; but clarification with the white of eggs is faster.

When no more feces precipitate, the water is distilled (in the water bath) and the residue carefully evaporated. The matter thus obtained is clear and red.

Now follows the preparation of the combustible oil and the Salarmeniac.

All former feces, including those of the white of eggs, are now distilled with strong firing at increasing temperatures. There must be some distilled water in the receiver. After about thirty hours of distillation, we use a feather to remove the bad-smelling oil floating on top. The oil is purified in distilled water; the water is added to the distillate.

The remaining liquid with the washing water of the oil is now distilled in the water bath, the distillate is poured upon the residue, the feces are filtered, and we distill again until the Salarmeniac is as white as snow.

Then follows the purification and rectification of the Earth. This, too, is done in the usual way through repeated distilling (coagulating), pouring back of the distillate, filtering of the feces, and another new distillation, till the Earth is quite white.

The white Earth is then dissolved in distilled water, the Salarmeniac is added to it, and the water is distilled to bone-dryness.

The residue is calcined in a flask in the laboratory furnace. With its own distilled water the whole mixture is now once again purified of the feces and coagulated. Now the Salarmeniac is ready to make the Stone.

Take the Fire, the Air, the Water, and the Earth and dissolve them in rectified water, coagulate again, put the matter once more into a flask, again calcine in the laboratory furnace. After this, it is again dissolved in distilled water, the feces are filtered, and we coagulate again. This is repeated until no more feces precipitate.

Now we put everything into a flask and pour only just as much water over it as is required for the solution. We now digest for twenty-four hours in the ash bath at summer temperature. Subsequently, we evaporate carefully until everything is dry (testing with a knife or mirror). Following this, we leave everything in the heat for three or four days.

Everything is now hermetically sealed and left for forty days in the athanor at a hot summer temperature.

After this, we let everything cool, remove the powder, put it into a glass crucible, and melt it. We then pour the Stone into a form coated with oil. While cooling, it will become hard, red, and transparent.

In this text Hollandus conceals certain things; he does not always express himself clearly. We must also read somewhat between the lines. In the author's experience, for instance, Salarmenia goes over easily. To get it, we have to catch it in the tubes during distillation and then quickly scratch it out.

Because of its enormous volatility, it is also called "eagle" in alchemy. Accordingly, we must build an eagle's trap with the tubes, in the hope that it gets stuck en route during distillation by precipitating on the glass wall.

The directions quoted are in no way simple recipes in the sense of cookbook instructions. The interested laboratory worker should first venture upon these works and remember that we learn as much from mistakes as from success. The pleasure of achieving will be twice as great if the Stone has been produced through one's own know-how.

Now follows Hollandus's text concerning the preparation of the Stone from honey.

How to Prepare Quintam Essentiam from Honey

Now I will reveal to you a great secret of the Vegetable Work, namely, the wonderful nature of honey, which is the subtlest and noblest of all plants and flowers, from whose purer and noble part it is elicited by the bees. For the nature of bees is such that they extract the best from them [plants and flowers], as has been reported in detail in the Animal-Work, where instructions are given on how to extract the nature of Animalia, especially described in chapter 84 of the Work. My child should know that everything God has created is extremely good, perfect, and imperishable, like heaven; but all things found here on earth, such as animals, fish, and whatever is sentient, as well as herbs, plants, and whatever it may be, have a double nature, that is, a perfect and an imperfect one. The perfect one is called Quinta Essentia; the imperfect one, however, the feces or the poisonous combustible oil. You must separate those feces and the combustible oil, and what then remains is perfect and is called Quinta Essentia. It lasts eternally like heaven and cannot be corrupted by anything, including fire. For when God had created everything and beheld it, everything was perfect and good, and nothing was lacking in anything. This I am telling you out of love: God has put a secret nature or influence into all created things, and a general influence into all of nature, and also a particular influence or virtue into every single species or genus, either regarding medicine or other secret effects, which are partly brought to light through natural art but are by far still more hidden than is known to our senses. Do you believe that a plant determined for this or that disease does not contain still other powers than those known to us? In truth, many more. I say, if the feces and the combustible oil, which is a poison in everything, causing death, are removed from this thing or that plant, and the Elements are purified and made to rise together over the alembic and are together united in one, it can afterward be a help and cure for all diseases, be it prepared from a plant, animal, or poison, as is shown in the preface to this book in chapter 14 and also in the preface to the Animal-Work, where instructions are given as to how to extract the Quinta Essentia from all, including poisonous animals, birds, worms, flies, and the like, and to bring them to a state where they can help the infirmities of all people. This can also especially be obtained from human blood, because with it it can best be proved that a person or an animal does not require any farfetched medicine for an accidental disease, for every animal has its own remedy for that disease. Without injuring a person or an animal, a medicament can be elicited from him or it with which the disease can be wonderfully cured, of which both the theory and the practice are taught there [in the two prefaces]. I only wished to insert this so that my child might understand what great wonders are contained in honey, which is taken from all flowers and gathered into one. Therefore, it must necessarily comprise various powers. For if God has infused into other things the power to heal, what will there be in honey, which is extracted from countless flowers, since each plant has its own gift? Truly, if one can bring it to its highest potency, it will operate wonderfully. Therefore, take note of what is hidden in this Quinta Essentia, so that you do not underestimate it but keep it secret as the most excellent of the whole Animal-Work. And when you have it, you do not require anything else for removing from the body anything bad befalling it.

Now I will pass to the practical work. Take 12 quarts of the best fresh virgin honey, put it into a big stone jar, put an alembic on it, lute [seal] it twice, set it in the Balneum and lute a receiver on it, let the Balneum boil, and distill as long as something rises. My child must know that there is no cloud-water in honey, only the Philosophical Elemental Water. The Element Air will first go over, together with the Element Fire, in which the Air is locked. The Air tastes like distilled Aqua Vitae and first ascends from the honey. Nor can it be distinguished from Aqua Vitae in looks or taste. Continue distilling until nothing rises any more. After this, let the jar with the alembic and receiver stay in the Balneum for 15 more days, the Balneum boiling all the time so that the matter may become quite dry, since the distillation of honey through the Balneum is very difficult on account of its fattiness. It must really stand in it for 15 or 20 days before it becomes quite dry. Now let it cool and take it out, detach the receptacle and alembic, and pour what is in the receptacle upon the dry matter. Set it in the Balneum, put on it a stopper or a piece of ground glass that fits well into the mouth of the jar, and seal it as well as possible—but the Balneum must only be lukewarm. In this way, my child, one could (and it would be a good thing) extract the Fire with its own Air, if one were willing to wait that long. It would also become much stronger, and the ancients did it in this way, but it is to be feared that the water would evaporate at the opening of the vessel, because it is subtle like wine, since the Air must each time it is drawn off be poured on again, and both the receptacle and the alembic must again be sealed on, and putrefaction must take place in the lukewarm Balneo. In the aforesaid way, the distillation must be repeated until all the Fire is out blood-red. However, in our times another way has been discovered, and that is as follows.

When, as said above, you have extracted all the Air and have completely dried the residual matter, take off the receptacle and stopper as well. Now have at hand rainwater distilled two or three times, pour a good amount of it—as much as you deem sufficient— into the jar, cover it, but do not seal it. Keep it in the boiling Balneo for three days and nights, stirred every day four or five times with a wooden spoon. Then let it cool, take it out, and let it settle. Now take another clean jar, pour the clear liquid off into it, again pour good distilled water on the feces as before, and again set the jar in the Balneum. Afterward, take it out and let it settle, pour the clear liquid off, and again pour a good portion of other distilled water on it, as before. Do this until the water no longer gets colored. Then you have got all the Fire out of the Earth. Preserve the Earth or feces until I teach you what to do with it, because it still contains the combustible oil.

Take the big stone jar containing all your colored water in addition to the Element Fire, distill all the water from it in the boiling Balneo, let it dry well and cool. Remove the alembic but leave the jar in the Balneo. Pour the water back on the matter, and stop up the mouth of the jar. Let the Balneum boil again, and keep the matter in it for three days, every day stirring it in the jar four or five times. Then let it cool, take it out of the Balneo, and let it settle. Now pour the clear liquid carefully off into a clean jar, and again pour fresh distilled water on the feces. Stir well, set it in the Balneum, let it once again settle for one day, pour the clear liquid off to the previous, and add the remaining feces to the others. Then put the jar back in the Balneum and distill the water off in the boiling Balneo until it becomes dry as before. Repeat this work until no more feces stay at the bottom. Put all the feces together with the previous Earth. Thus you have the Element Fire quite pure. After this, the Element Air must also be distilled over until no feces remains in fundo vitri. Then you have the Element pure. At last, draw the Fire off from the water and dry it, and you will have a transparent Massa, or a clear red matter, shining like camphor. Preserve the Fire in a clean glass jar, and keep the Air with the water well closed in a glass until you have also prepared the Earth.

Take therefore all the Earth with the fecibus and extract its combustible oil per descensum by means of two containers, one sealed upon the other. One of them must be dug into the earth, but on the other a fire must be made as long as the oleum combustible goes off. This oil is used for cold weaknesses and other diseases that would take too long to mention here. But if you do not want this oleum, let it go; it is not worth much.

Take the Earth and calcine it quite gently in the reverberating furnace until it becomes white as snow. Then put it into a big stone jar, pour upon it a sufficient quantity of distilled common water, stir it with a wooden spoon, set it in the boiling Balneum for three days, stirring it every day ten or twelve times. Now let it cool, remove the jar, and let it stand for one day until it settles. Then pour the clear carefully off into another clean container and again pour more distilled water on the feces, and keep it in the Balneo as before. Remove it again and let it stand for one day and one night, and once more pour the clear liquid off gently into the previous. Repeat this imbiding and decanting a third time. When that is done, pour the feces out, for they are no longer of any use. After this, take the jar with all the water poured together, set it in the boiling Balneum, distill it to total dryness, let it cool, then again pour the water over the Earth or Salt, and keep it dissolving in the boiling Balneo. After this, let it cool and sink, pour the clear liquid off into another jar, and again some distilled water on the feces. Set it for three or four hours in the hot Balneum, remove it again, and let it settle for a few hours. Then gradually pour the clear liquid off on top into the first and throw the feces out, for there is nothing left in them. After this, set the jar with the Earth or Salt back in the Balneum, draw off the water until quite dry, and proceed in everything as before. Repeat this operation until no more feces remain at the bottom. Now extract the water from the Earth, and you will find it [the Earth] beautiful and clear like a crystal, and thus you will have your Element pure.

Thereupon, in God's name, take a large glass that can stand the fire. Pour your Earth and Fire into it, and pour the Air upon it. Put that glass on a furnace in a cupel with ashes, firmly lute [seal] an alembic on it with a hole on top instead of a button, so that the water, after it has been completely distilled, can again be imbibed through a funnel. It has to be drawn off each time to a pint. Then, first, start a small fire under it, which you must make stronger by and by until you see the matter boil through the glass. Now keep it thus boiling at an even temperature until it is distilled off to a pint. Then let the fire in the furnace go out, and let it cool. Afterward remove the receiver, open the hole in the alembic, mount a glass funnel on it, and through it pour all the water in the receptacle on the Earth. Lute again, and again distill the water over as before, and repeat this ten times. Hereafter, distill everything over, because the Earth has become volatile after the tenth distillation. Consequently, the Air, the Water, the Fire, and the Earth rise simultaneously through the alembic as one substance, and those which before were four have now become a single one in nature and are now simple like the imperishable heaven. They are not yet fixed, however, but conjoined in such a way that they cannot be separated but will eternally remain a simple Corpus like a crystal or like that indestructible heaven. What do you think, my child: should the Quinta Essentia not be able to drive away all diseases that may befall man because of their high temperature, be it a disease due to heat, cold, humidity, or dryness? Everything is in it, to give to each what is required, like heaven, which, when the earth requires cold, warmth, moisture, or dryness, gives it all to it, and yet it is neither warm, cold, moist, nor dry but a simple essence and endowed with such a nature that it can give to each what he needs. Likewise with this Quinta Essentia. Therefore, my son, rejoice and thank the Lord who has given the knowledge of it to the philosophers.

Now, my child, if you wish to bring this Quinta Essentia to great perfection, take a big circulating glass or pelican, which is a glass with a big head like an alembic. In the upper point of it there must be a hole, so that the matter can be poured into it with a funnel and the hole immediately closed tightly. From the head two crooked arms go to the belly, and that which then rises flows back into the belly through the arms. The "pelican" has the shape of a glass that drives substances up and down within itself—it looks like a pelican [bird]. Therefore, take the Quinta Essentia, put it into the Pelican, distill on sifted ashes or, better, on dry prepared salt, light a fire that is warm like the summer heat, and the Quinta Essentia will rise in the form of a red oil, and will again descend through the arms of the glass, and will become even thicker through frequent ascending and descending until it finally stays at the bottom and no longer rises.

Now increase the fire to make the Quinta Essentia rise and fall again, and keep the fire at the same grade until it no longer ascends but stays below. Then increase the fire to make it rise and fall once more, and keep that same grade of heat until it stays below. Observe such an increase of the fire carefully until the matter becomes fixed.

When the Quinta Essentia no longer rises, it is fixed and brought to the highest virtue. Remove it from the glass while it is still warm. Otherwise, if you let it grow cold and hard, you would have to break the glass. It melts in the heat and becomes hard when cold. It penetrates everything hard as oil does dry leather; its color is ruby-red and like a transparent crystal; it glows in the dark enough to read by its light.

What do you think of it, my child? Has God not created wonderful bodies? In truth, he has not endowed the philosophers with lesser gifts so that they can see that which is hidden in nature. This medicine has an unbelievable effect, because, as it consists of the subtlest of all plants, trees, flowers, and blossoms of fruits from which the little bees gathered it when the herbs and trees were in bloom, it may rightly be called Lapis Philosophorum. It is fixed and fusable like wax. Like the Mineral Stone which transmutes imperfect metals into ☉ and ☽, this Stone changes all diseases into health. From this it is evident that honey has preference among all vegetable things. However, as long as it is still in its impure and crude form, it is hardly suitable for medicines. No matter how much it is boiled and skimmed, it nevertheless keeps its nature, because it consists of various earthy growths, plants, and trees: one is hot, the other cold, the third dry, the fourth moist, the fifth stopping, the sixth driving, the seventh pungent, the eighth poisonous, and so forth. Each has its own quality. That is why honey is good for one infirmity and harmful for another. For each acts according to its property when the separation is done in the body, and from that comes the blood and other humors. It can be compared to gunpowder, which does not do any harm as long as it lies still, but as soon as it gets together with fire, it shows its hidden power and burns with a fierce fire that cannot be extinguished with water. Because of the quarrel among cold, heat, moisture, and dryness, there occurs such a bang and wind that it shatters everything close to it.

Likewise with honey. When it reaches the region of the liver, in order to separate, it shows there its nature by puffing up violently, so that it would not be surprising if such a quarrel would cause the veins of the liver to rupture, as happens sometimes. That is the reason why abcesses develop at various places. Honey causes such puffing that the veins can easily burst from it. And although there are many who extol it with great praise, they are nevertheless no sons of philosophy, nor do they understand nature. But when honey is brought to a simple, fixed essence, it is the highest medicine among the Vegetabilia, like wine, so that nothing like it can be found in the world. Thank God and be good to the poor. The dose is one grain, to be taken in the morning on an empty stomach and every day at night, until the end of the sickness. All infirmities are cured by it, just as the Mineral Stone makes projection on metals. Praise God and work diligently.

Summary of the Processes

Honey is distilled to dryness in the water bath, when the Elements Air and Fire go over first (it requires much time, fifteen to twenty days). The Air tastes like Aqua Vitae.

The distillate is poured back; the flask is closed and set in a lukewarm bath. The Element Fire is now extracted with its own Air. The distillation is repeated until all the Fire is out blood-red.

Another way: After the Air has been drawn off to dryness (to be kept till later!) the residue is washed with rainwater three times distilled. (Dissolve in the boiling water bath.) We let the feces precipitate, the liquid is decanted, more distilled water is poured on the feces, again we extract through the water bath, let the feces precipitate, and decant the liquid. This process is repeated until there is no more coloring.

The liquids are then poured together.

Now the Fire Element is rectified.

The colored water is distilled to dryness in the water bath. We let the feces precipitate, pour the liquid off, add new distilled water upon the feces, and extract again. The resulting liquid is added to the first; the feces are added to the Earth. The extracted liquid is distilled, poured back, the feces filtered, and so on, until everything is pure. The Fire-Salt is then evaporated in the water bath through evaporation.

Now the combustible oil is distilled from the Earth and the fecibus; it does not become part of the work. The Earth is washed out of the residue with distilled water (let it stand in the water bath for three days), the solution is decanted, further extracted with fresh distilled water, again decanted, and the feces are extracted yet a third time, after which we throw them out.

The Earth-Salt and the Fire-Salt are now put into a flask, the Air extracted in the beginning is poured on them, and the liquid is distilled in the ash bath to one pint. (The matter in the fractionating flask is boiling.)

Ten cohobations now follow; the distillate is therefore poured back each time and again distilled. In this way the Earth becomes volatile and rises over with the rest. (Cf. the Circulatum Minus.)

Now everything is rotated in the pelican at a temperature equal to the heat of the summer sun. When no more matter rises, we increase the heat until it again stays below.

We increase the fire until the matter remains fixed. After this, we heat once more strongly for twenty-four hours until the Quinta Essentia (the Stone) no longer rises.

As long as the Stone is still warm, we can take it out of the pelican; it will get hard in the cold. We can either cast or mold the Stone. It has a red color and is transparent and fluorescent. We can also let the Stone get hard in the pelican or the congealing glass, and then break the glass to remove the Stone.

Finally, there now follows a slightly simplified form of the *Opus*

Vini, the work with wine. The text stems from the famous collection *Aureum Vellus or Gulden Schatzkammer* (1598; Hamburg edition, 1718). The *Golden Vlies* has also been published by the Akademische Druck- und Verlagsanstalt in Graz, Austria, under the title *Schatzkammer der Alchemie.*

Tractatus de Quinta Essentia Vini

First, in the Name of God, take clear Rhine wine or other fine, clear wine drawn from the mother [a thick sediment in wine], because there must not be any impurity in it, as the philosophers say that we must draw our Stone from one thing without adding anything foreign to it. Therefore, take good, clear wine, good of smell and taste. Separate its four Elements as much as possible, because it is impossible to separate the Elements perfectly, that is, to extract simultaneously the Air from the Fire. That is impossible, as the Air is hot and moist. Consequently, the moisture cannot be perfectly separated from the heat. Water is cold and moist, and therefore we cannot separate the cold from the moist perfectly. Likewise the Fire. It is hot and dry, therefore we cannot separate the heat from dryness. Accordingly, it is impossible to separate the Elements simultaneously, but they must first be and remain mixed together, because in every Element there are two natures, one manifest, the other secret.

Exemplum: Water is cold and moist. The moisture is manifest, the cold is secret and invisible, and is a soul without a body, and is hidden under the moisture. The Air is hot and moist. The moisture is manifest and visible; the heat, however, is a spirit and secret. Fire is hot and dry and clear, and is both subtle and spiritual. The clearness and redness are manifest, the heat is secret as dryness, for if you see a light burn, you will well see the clearness and redness from outside with your eyes, but you cannot see the heat that the fire has within. Yet put a finger into the light and you will feel the invisible heat. The Earth is cold and dry. Its dry body is visible and tangible, but its coldness is invisible and is a spirit without a body.

It is therefore evident that it is impossible to separate the Elements, but they must be mixed together—and yet we must do it as much as possible. We can separate them, as we shall see later, and rectify them of their imperfection, and can make them so pure, beautiful, hard, and fixed when they are united that we can never again separate them, and they will in all eternity be a clarified Corpus that cannot be consumed by fire.

Aristotle says in a little book he has written that everything on earth has two natures, one secret, the other evident. That which appears by nature on the outside has its contrarium inside. That which is hot and dry outside is moist and cold inside. Let us therefore see how we can reverse all things and bring their inside outside, and vice versa; then we can achieve a perfect work. And this must be done from one single thing without adding anything foreign to it.

That is why Aristotle says: When you have the Water from the Air, and the Air from the Fire, and the Fire from the Earth, and have separated them perfectly from every impurity, you have the right Art, and out of it comes a Stone, and it is no stone and not of the nature of a stone, but an eternally perfect body, lasting in all eternity. And this is the secret that God has left to the world. Therefore, take fine, good, clear wine, the best in smell and taste. Put it into a big stone jar, containing about 16 or 20 Mass [quarts]. Put an alembic on it and lute [seal] it tightly, set it in B.M. [Balneum Mariae, or water bath], add a receptacle, and distill with gentle heat, in six stages, as slowly as the clock strikes. When you see a small drop appear inside the alembic, like dew, remove the receptacle and take the jar out of the B. Now have ready another jar, the bigger the better. Put your Air [distillate] into it, set the alembic on the jar, lute it very well, attach a receptacle, distill it with a lukewarm fire in six stages, and continue distilling it thus in this heat until you see the dew come into the alembic. Then remove the receptacle, close it well, lute another receptacle in front, carefully attached to the tubes of the alembic. Distill until you notice a clear thin water coming out.

Now take this receptacle, plug it up with wax, remove the alembic from the jar, and pour what is still in the jar into the first water which you had first retained. Clean your jar thoroughly, dry it with a nice linen cloth so that no moisture remains in it. Then pour that which you drew off last back into it, again put the alembic on the jar, well luted as before, until you can again see the dew appear in the alembic.

Then stop. Remove the lid of the receptacle, pour what is left in the jar into the first water you have drawn off. Cleanse your jar with a linen cloth, pour all the Air you have collected back into the jar, again attach the alembic, distill in the same heat as I have taught before until you see some dew come into the alembic. Then remove the receptacle, put another one on, distill until almost everything has gone over, then remove the alembic and pour what is left in the jar to the first water.

Now take a fine glass, put into it all the Air you have, attach an alembic, distill it in the B. with the same heat as has been taught before. Repeat the distillation until nothing remains at the bottom of the glass and there is no dew above in the alembic. Take what is in the glass port at the bottom and add everything to the first water. When everything goes over clear—what is in the glass port stays as it was when you poured it in—and you see no more dew come into the alembic, you have rectified the Air. Put it into a glass phial, stop it well with wax, and preserve it until you need it.

Now take your jar still containing the water, put an alembic on, set it in the B., and distill it with a small fire in the third degree, until the matter becomes dry. When you see that nothing will distill anymore, increase the fire under the B.M. to make the water boil strongly, and keep it thus boiling for twenty-four hours, so that if some Fire had remained with the Fire and the Earth, the same could all be drawn off nicely. When you see that nothing is distilled anymore, no matter how strongly the B.M. is boiling, stop, let it cool, and remove the receptacle. Now take a nice jar and pour all the water into it, but remove the jar with the water and the Earth from the B. Take the alembic off and put it on the jar into which you have poured all your waters. Set it in the B., distill with a gentle fire, so that you might count to six between every drop falling from the tubes of the alembic. Distill thus until it no longer drips, then increase the fire under the B. to boiling for four to five hours. When you then see that it no longer drips, stop, and do not distill any-more. Let it cool.

Take the receptacle and the alembic off. Remove what you find at the bottom of the jar and add it to the other Fire and Earth which were left after the first distillation. Wash the jars well and then pour all your water back into them, attach the alembic, set it back in the B., put the receptacle in front, distill it again with a small fire, as said before. When it no longer drips, let it cool, remove the recep-tacle with all your water, and take the alembic off the jar. Again, add what you find at the bottom to the Fire and Earth. Clean the jar again, dry it well with a linen cloth, and once more pour all your waters into it, put the alembic on, and distill again as before.

You must continue with this distillation until nothing is left at the bottom of the jar, but until everything goes over as nicely as you had put it in and the jar stays just as nice. Take it out, remove the receptacle, pour all your water into a phial or stone jar, stopper it well with wax, and set it aside until you need it. Now you have your Air and your Fire, each by itself, in a separate container, rectified and rid of all their humoribus.

Now let us see further and separate the Fire and Earth. First, remove all the Fire together with the Earth from the jar, and put it all into a big earthenware container well luted—everything together, so that nothing will stay behind. After this, take some roof tiles. Burn those in a strong fire for an hour or two, then let them cool. Pulver-ize them, sift them through a small sieve, mix this powder, the Fire and also the Earth in the cupel, enough to dry them to powder. If you wish to mix this powder, you must put the cupel on a tripod and light a fire underneath to heat the matter. Otherwise you will not be able to mix much of the powder. When that has been done, take an earthenware barrel, put the matter into it, add the alembic, then lute it so well that it can stand the fire.

The barrel, however, should now be one-third full, so that two-thirds remain. Set the barrel on a furnace, with a cupel filled with ashes, put a receptacle in front, lute the Earth well, because the Fire is a subtle spirit. Then light a fire in the furnace, very gently for the first four hours, the next four somewhat stronger, the third four hours still stronger, while during the last four the cupel with the matter must be red-hot. Keep it this way until nothing will distill over anymore. When you notice that, let it stand thus in the flame for about another hour. You must let it glow carefully, because it would not be good for the Earth if it became white (while it is still closed).

When it has stood red-hot for one hour, let it cool after it has stopped dripping. Remove the receptacle, likewise the alembic and the water, and you will find at the bottom a black substance like coal, which is a precious Stone, and it is the blood of the Earth. Take it out and preserve it well until you need it.

In the receptacle, however, there is a thick black substance, vel terra. In it there is the Fire, but it is impure and still has with it some of the Element Earth. Now take a stone jar, put into it one part of the clarified water. Distill three times as much water as there is Fire. Put the Fire and water together into the jar, take a wooden spoon with a long handle, and mix the water and Fire for one or two hours without stop, stirring well. Then lute an alembic on it with Luto sapientiae to make it fireproof, set it in ashes, and first give it a gentle fire until the jar gets warm; then increase the fire so much that it comes out of the tubes of the alembic.

Keep it thus in the fire, in the third grade, until nothing will distill over, or increase the fire for one hour to see if something will still rise. Then you will have the Water and the Fire well mixed together. Now remove the alembic and add that which you find at the bottom to your Earth.

Now take a fine jar, put your Water and Fire into it, distill in the B., enough to count six between drops. Then the Water will go over and the Fire stay at the bottom. Remove the jar from the B., set it in ashes, distill over, add what stays at the bottom to the Earth. Once again, take the Water with the Fire, pour it again into the jar, stir it for one hour with a spoon, so that it gets well mixed. Then add an alembic, set it again in the ashes as before, distill until nothing goes over, and then distill again out of the B.

Repeat this kind of distillation until nothing more goes over but everything comes out as beautifully as you had poured in it. After each distillation, add everything that stays behind to the first Earth. But when nothing stays behind any longer, then it is enough, and then your Fire is perfectly separated from its Earth. Then it is red, clear, and subtler than the Air. Pour that Fire into a glass phial and stop it well with wax. Now your Fire is well rectified and separated from all its earthiness, and it is pure. In this way you have all three, Air, Fire, and Water, perfect for accomplishing your Work in them.

Now let us see further and change the black Earth into a crystalline Stone, and separate the black Earth, thus completing our Work. Take all the black Earth, pulverize it in a mortar, and sift it through a small sieve. After this, take five or six earthenware pans with a flat bottom and a port one thumb high. Into the bottom of this pan put your Earth, half a finger's thickness, set it in a reverberating furnace and calcine it until it is enough.

Keep it for twelve hours in red heat, but only so that it may glow and no more. Then let it cool and remove the pan with the Earth. Have at hand a nice stone or glass jar, but a stone jar is better. Pulverize all your earth and sift it through a sieve, put it into the jar, take water from your receptacle, and pour it upon the Earth. Stir it well with a wooden spoon with a long handle.

Now set the jar in the Balneum, put something over the mouthpiece, light a fire under the B., so that the water becomes so hot that you cannot put your hand in it. Stir it every hour with the spoon, and let it stand in this heat for 12 hours. Then let it cool and decrease the fire day and night. Thereafter take another stone jar and pour the clear water off the fecibus or draw it per filtrum through a cloth, as you know how to do. Then once more pour your rectified aqua upon the feces of the Earth. Stir it again with the spoon, set it in the Balneum, and do as before. After this, let it be clarified as before, again, pour the clear off per filtrum, and add it to the other water which you drew off first.

Thereafter, take the jar with the aqua in which your Earth is dissolved, and the alembic, set it in the B., and distill the water over. Then the Earth will stay at the bottom of the jar as a gray salt. Take that out, pulverize it, and put it back into the pan, as is said above. Set it in the reverberating furnace, give it a gentle fire so that it glows moderately, as before, and let it stand in the flame for two hours. Watch the Earth carefully to prevent it from melting; otherwise it will be all spoiled.

That is why the fire has to burn gently, just as if you wished to perforate an iron. Otherwise the Earth would melt, become spoiled, so that it would afterward not go out during distillation. Therefore, do not burn it too hot, so that it will not melt. Then let it cool, remove it from the pan, pulverize it subtly, and put it back into the jar. Pour the Rectified Water upon it, stir it with the spoon, set it in the fire, make the B. hot, let it stand for 12 hours, stirring it every hour with the spoon. After this, let it cool, also stand day and night, and settle.

Then pour the clear liquid off above into another jar and filter it. Again pour more Rectified Water on the feces, stir, and set it back in the B. as before. When it is done, pour it into the previous, put the alembic back on the jar, and set it in the B. Distill the aqua from the Earth with a small fire, and your Earth will stay at the bottom of the jar and should be quite white. Now remove the Earth from the jar and pulverize it or rub it on a stone to a subtle powder. Put it back into the pan, reverberate it as before, first with a small fire to let it glow sweetly without getting a taste, and do not let it stand in the flame longer than you can say three or four Paternosters.

After this, let it cool, and remove the pan, again rub the Earth on a stone to a pure powder, put it back into the jar, pour your Rectified Water back on it, stir, set it again in the B., and proceed further as mentioned above. Do not leave any feces in your powder. You must coagulate, distill, decant, and calcine. When now the Earth is dissolved, it is pure, well rectified, and white as snow. Now you have the four Elements, each rectified by itself. Therefore, rejoice, because you are now ready to complete your Work.

Now we shall see how the Elements can again be brought together, to make of them a perfect Corpus lasting eternally. You must know that the perfection of the Stone and the Art lies in the Earth, for Hermes Philosophus says: "In the earth lies the perfection of all works, for without the earth no thing can be perfect, because the earth is solid and the fixation of all perfection, and without the earth no thing can be congealed and no thing can get any power except from the earth, and you should know that the earth is very small but has great powers."

One can see many grains spring from a small grain. Take great care that you now do not take anything foreign but its own Earth. For there are some who believe that they are making aquam vitae while they are making aquam mortis. The reason is that they take foreign Earth, saying that it is its own Earth. Others take the wine from the winepress with the grapes and small stones and say that it is a perfect Earth. Still others take the vine, which they burn to ashes, making a lye of it, which they coagulate, saying it is terra vini. But all of them are mistaken, and believing that they are making aquae vitae, they make aquae mortis. But the Physici say that you must make something from a thing that is perfect and that you must not add anything foreign to it. But if you use grapes from the winepress that are not perfect for man's necessities of life and extract the Elements from them, as has been taught above, the Earth which will then remain is its own Earth and not a foreign one.

Exemplum: When the wine comes out of the winepress, it is rotten and not clear, its feces and dregs are at the bottom, and it ferments every spring. Its tartar leaves it and adheres to the sides of the vat, and that, too, is nothing but feces. Thus the wine casts off all feces and bad humors above and below at the bottom, likewise from all sides. When it becomes clear and beautiful and has cast off all feces, it also acquires a good smell and taste and is very pleasant to drink and take. And then it is *one* thing.

But as long as it still has with it some feces or some turbidity, it is not *one* thing, since it still contains that which must leave it before it becomes pleasant and clear. From this it is evident that one should take neither tartar, grapes, nor wine from the winepress or dregs, nor use the ashes of vine, since they all have bad humors which the wine casts off before it becomes fit to drink. Those who content themselves with such works are altogether mistaken, believing that they make aquam vitae while they are making aquam mortis, because they take an imperfect thing which the wine repels by nature before it becomes fit to drink. This is just as if a physician were to take many bad humors and substances of which he rids a man and would then try to cure another sick person with the same bad, rotten substance. Thus it is with those who hold such opinions about foreign Earth.

Therefore, the Physici say: Our Stone must be made from one thing, and nothing foreign must ever be added to it. Consequently, it is clear and true, because of the aforesaid reasons, that one should take beautiful, clear wine and make of it aquam vitae to preserve man's life, not to become corrupted to his last day by some accidental humors, and to restore us to the first state of health.

Why have I said this? To put you on guard against foreign Earth, and because of the ignorant ones who are trying to put other fantasies into your heads, and to take you off the path of error so that you should at all times stay on the right road without error. Also, if you do take foreign Earth, you will not know how much of the foreign Earth you should or must take in proportion to the Air. Therefore, stay with the prescribed Regulis.

You must also know that you must not take the Element Fire in any medicine, because it is too hot. It will consume and destroy the natural moisture of man's body, because the life of all men and animals rests on two things, that is, on warmth and moisture, and the better those are tempered, the stronger and healthier the nature is.

Therefore, do not take the Element Fire for any medicinal work. The Air is hot and moist, the Earth cool and dry, and with the cold of the Earth you must temper the heat of the Air, and then achieve a Quintam Essentiam or a clarified Corpus and the Lapidem Philosophorum. When it is done, reflect well of what complexion or nature it is and what is enclosed in it when the Earth and the Air are congealed together and turned into a crystal, and whether it is also a protection in the heat, and whether it adjusts to the cold. And if it were standing in the fire for a hundred years, its essence and nature would not change, nor would it lose any of its weight. Read this lesson over frequently, and then you will yourself discover of what complexion the Stone is and what can be achieved with it.

But to return to our work and propositum of marrying and joining the Elements. So take, in the name of the Lord, all your Rectified Earth, put it into a glass vat, pour upon it some of your Rectified Water, just enough to dissolve your Earth and no more, and this is to take place in the Balneum. When your Earth is dissolved into clear water, take a glass with an alembic on top, and pour your dissolved Earth into it. You should know that you must not pour more water upon it than is necessary to dissolve it. When you have put your Earth into the glass, pour your Air upon it and shake them well together by hand. Then put the glass, well stoppered on top, in a B. and let it stand in it for four or five days. Now take it out and place it on a furnace in ashes, lute an alembic on it, and attach a receptacle. Distill first with a gentle fire, then gradually stronger, continuing thus until nothing distills anymore. Then let it cool, and your Earth will remain at the bottom of the vat. Remove it, pulverize it on a stone with wine of your Rectified

Water. Powder it so small and subtle that one could paint with it with a brush. Now return your powdered Earth to the glass, again pour the Air upon it, stir it well, and set it back in the B., well stopped up, for four or five days, stirring once every day to mix it well. Then set it again in ashes and again distill per alembicum, as mentioned before.

Repeat such a distillation until the Earth is completely distilled over. Take note: there is still another way to distill the Earth, which is less work. When now the Earth has gone over, it is as the Physicus says: the lowest must be like the highest, or else no coniunctio or conjoining will take place, because the Earth must be made spiritual.

Therefore, all wise men say, make the lowest like the highest, and the highest like the lowest, then you have a stable work well done. And if the Earth were made volatile and the Air fixed, but the Earth did not go over with the Air, they could never unite or congeal, for when they distill over together, they grasp each other fundamentally, and there results such a union that they will never separate. It will remain an eternal coniunctio, just as it will be with our body and soul after Judgment Day, because there will be no mixture of the Elements, but they will become one single being, a Simple Essence, a one-thing essence, like heaven, which contains the four Elements without being mixed, because they are simple and *one*. That is how heaven holds the four Elements.

Still more is it *one* in our work, because the Earth has now left and is distilled over with the Air, and they are united in such a way that they can never again be separated, and although nothing has yet been congealed, there is nothing between the Elements, because they are equally divided. In regard to the Air, it was hot and humid, the Earth was cold and dry, and as much moisture as the Air has too much, as much moisture was lacking in the Earth, and thus its dryness is tempered with the moisture of the Air. And as much heat as the Air has too much, as much cold there is in the Earth, and the Earth is tempered with the heat of the Air. The Air is very light, spiritual, and volatile; the Earth is heavy, corporeal, and fixed. Now mark what unity there is between the Air and the Earth.

The two opposites, which are now conjoined, have grasped each other fundamentally so much that they flew up together out of the cucurbit into the heaven of the alembic, and have become *one* thing. Therefore, ask your understanding what kind of a thing it might be, whether it does not have in itself the four Elements, and if they are not evenly divided as said before, and if they are not beautifully clear and pure on account of the separation and rectification, which have been taught before, and if they are not rightly conjoined, since they went up together through the alembic. Think of this lesson and remember it well, for here hidden Secreta and concealed things are revealed which had always been withheld by the alchemists of old.

Therefore, thank and praise God Almighty for His wonder work and holy gifts He has given to His dear philosophers, because in this work all other Secreta are included, just as the door to all secrets is here opened to you. Accordingly, do not spare any pains studying this, to enable you to pass through the door into the domum Philosophorum, so that you may see this wondrous thing. Now enough of that.

Now let us see how we can fix these four Elements which have been distilled through the alembic, make them eternal, and bring them to their highest power. Take then, in the name of the Holy Trinity, the substance in the receptacle, pour it into the fixing glass and close it with Sigillo Hermetis, set it in cineris or ashes, not deeper than the substances is, and give it a small fire for the first eight days, then increase the fire for the next eight days when the matter begins to become coarse and ascend slowly. That you must see and notice! The matter comes and rises from the bottom of that vat into the head and descends again. Then you will see many small veins rise from the head of the glass and go down to the bottom, of which veins there are very many and innumerable ones because of their subtlety.

Now, however, the streamlets will become somewhat thicker through the ascending and descending. When they begin to get thicker, there will be fewer than before when they were quite subtle. At this stage you must increase the fire somewhat, because your matter is about to become fixed. For the thicker and coarser the small veins become, the fewer there are of them, and the more fixed the matter becomes, the better it can stand the fire. This is the sign to increase your fire until you see that no more veins rise and descend in the glass. After this, you must keep the matter in the same heat for eight days, when you will see another sign of which the philosophers write so wonderfully, and it is a sign of perfection.

For Aristotle speaks: *De Secretis Secretorum,* chapter 15: "Our Water is no water or pouring of water. It is our instrument and hammer, gauge, file, or plane, with which we must work just as a blacksmith must forge the iron with the hammer if he is to bend it to his will. And when the iron has been hammered in accordance with the master's will, he hangs it on the wall. Or the carpenter works with the plane, but when the work is done, the plane does not stay with the work and is hung on the wall.

Likewise it is with our work, even more so, because the cloud-water is the hammer or plane with which we achieve our work, for with the cloud-water we must disengage or dissolve our work; with it we must also extract and separate the Elements. And when we have separated them, we must wash them with cloud-water, just as a woman washes her linen. When it is washed, she hangs it in the sun and no longer continues to wash. Look at the cloth dyers. If they wish to dye cloth or garments, they cannot get the color into the cloth without cloud-water. They must prepare the dye with water and boil it on fire without the cloth. When the cloth is dyed, they hang it up to dry. The water dries up, and the color stays fixed in the cloth.

Likewise with our work, for with water we have completed our work, fixed our Stone, and we now no longer require water. Now think how you purged the Air and the Earth. First you dissolved the Earth in Rectified Fire, which you had first drawn from your work per distillationem, and you rubbed your Earth twice or three times on the stone with your water, and the work has thus been accomplished, thanks to God, and this water does *not* belong to the Lapide Philosophorum.

Because it is water of the clouds, it is our harbor and gauge, and we have not worked in vain since the Stone has been accomplished. When it is fixed, you will see this sign: at the place where you previously saw the small veins rise and descend from the bottom of the vat to the head above, you will now see drops in the head all over the glass, and they will fall back again on the fixam Materiam. Just as the dew drips from the leaves upon the earth, so it happens here. When you see this sign, rejoice, because the Stone of Life is accomplished and the Q.E. achieved in the way it can be prepared by human hands. It is the supreme medicine that God has left in nature, because it has the power to drive away all infirmities and to purge man to enable him to live without diminution to his last day. What else it can do, I do not disclose, for those who understand the work well know what miracles it can perform. That I leave to those who will understand.

When you notice the last signs, let your fire die out and the glass cool down. When it is cool, you will find a hard Stone at the bottom of the water, while the water is standing above the Stone. Know, if there were no water and the Stone were beginning to become fixed, it would pass through the glass like oil through dry leather.

Therefore, let the glass first cool down well before you pour off the water, because the water keeps the Stone from penetrating through the glass, for as long as the glass is clean, the Stone is molten, since it dissolves in hot, dry air and coagulates in cold, moist air. Therefore, let it cool down very well.

When the water is out, break the glass and remove the King of Eternity, who will always preserve his crown and power, and thank Almighty God for His holy gifts, etc.

Now has been accomplished what has been solemnly promised. Our Stone must be made, the Physici say, out of *one* thing, without adding anything foreign to it, and it should contain the four Elements—which has been sufficiently taught and proved by explanations and speeches. That is why Hermes says: "You should not open your purse and incur great expense." And Arnoldus de Villanova says in "Novo Testamento": "The Lord God has given us two Stones, one to the White and one to the Red, which we can have without pay, as they grow, and one can have of them as much as one wishes, and we need not ask anybody's permission. And whoever knows this Stone and can prepare it, will not have much expense with the Art."

Therefore, remember well what I have here shown you, I have opened the door for you. Enter joyfully the house of the philosophers, and start working with your little understanding. Then you will see and understand wonderful things. By frequently reading this lesson over before you begin to work, no harm will befall your work, because I have told and written everything clearly, without any veiled words, and I have opened for you the way that I have gone with great care and labor, and I have rid you of your worry and work. I have also warned you of all accidents and errors that you might encounter in the work, without obscure words or words mixed with wrong advice, so that you should get a clear understanding without losing any time. If you had previously understood differently, you can now much better understand from this work that I have described to you, for what has to be done in the Art must all aim at one way and path, or else it will end in great expense and fantasy, and one will thus become the laughingstock of all men.

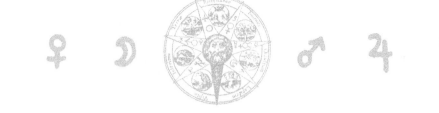

12
ALCHEMICAL SIGNS AND SYMBOLS

P rior to the standardization of scientific and technical concepts in our time, every art had its own signs and symbols; thus the corresponding texts were only accessible to initiates. This was done to prevent abuses by unauthorized persons.

There now follows a list of the most important signs commonly used in plant alchemy, which facilitates the deciphering of old texts even at an advanced stage of learning.

Of what elements are the signs formed?

Part of the signs consist of the initial letters of the corresponding Latin terms.

For example: $\mathcal{B}$ = Lat. *balneum* = bath; $\mathcal{G}$ = Lat. *gutta* = drop; $\mathcal{CC}$ = Lat. *cornum cervi* = hartshorn, etc.

Another group represents combinations of initials with symbols, for instance, $\mathcal{A}$ = to draw off, to decant; $V\!3$ = Lat. *vaporis balneum* = steam (vapor) bath; $\mathcal{QE}$ = Lat. *tartarus emeticus* = tartar emetic; $\frown$ = *spiritus*.

The sign $\frown$, or combinations with it, frequently point to volatile substances or processes of volatilization, such as $\mathcal{D}$ = to distill; $\mathcal{F}$ = to digest, strictly speaking, to digest through circulation; $\widehat{c}$ = to calcine (when substances become volatile); $\overline{V}$ means the alcoholic life water (Aqua Vitae); and $\mathcal{F}$ means fire grade (when substances rise). The sign

━᠕᠊ itself may mean: spirit, to anneal, to calcine, to sublimate, mineral turpentine (old name Turpeth), etc.

A reversal of the sign frequently indicates the contrary of volatile, for example, $\widetilde{HE}$ = crystal; ═᠊᠊᠊═ = precipitate, especially white precipitate, and also precipitated.

On the other hand, ━᠊°᠊━ means year; ═᠊°᠊═ pound; ═᠊᠊᠊═, ─᠊᠊᠊─, or ═᠊᠊᠊᠊ instead, spirit.

It is therefore always essential to pay attention to the right context.

Part of the symbols represent the things themselves, for example, ♤ = glass; ░░░ = sand; ≈ = water; ℘ = to distill (to bring over the alembic); ✡ = Elements, composed of △, ▽, ◬, and ⍟; ⍫ means filtering, etc.

Typical are also the many abbreviations: Rhab. = rhubarb (from the German *Rhabarber*); Sem. = Lat. *semen* = seed; Col. = Lat. *colaturae* = to percolate; S. et. C. = *simplex et compositum* = simple and compound; q.p. = *quantum placet* = as much as desired; Spec. = *Species* = species.

Reading old texts and familiarizing oneself with the alchemical terminology and symbolism belong to the most fascinating adventures of the study. But only long experience and the ability to view all details synoptically when studying old texts can shed light on the matter.

Add *add* .

Air △ , ⚖ , ꓱ , # .

Alembic ꞏ .

Alembic, distilling ⅩⅩ , ⅩⅩ , ꝫ , ꙮ .

Anneal; calcine (v.) ⌐ , ⌐ , ⌐ .

Aqua Vitae ꙮ , ⚹ , Ⅴ , ♅ , ♅ , Ⅳ , ☿ , ♏ .

Aquarius ≈ .

Aries ♈ .

As much as remains *q.l.*

Ash ⣿ , ⬩ , Ɛ , ♀ , A , E , ⌐ .

Ash-salt Ц , ♄ , ♏ , Λ , ꙮ , θ , ⊔ , 8 , ℱ , R .

Autumn ♎ , 20 , ⊖ , ⚋ .

Basic parts of bodies ♁ , ♂ , ⚷ , ✡ .

Bath B₊ , ℬ .

Bath, vapor (steam) V , V3 ,

Bath, water MB , ℳB , BM , ▽ꝛ , ℬ .

Blind flask △ , ◇ , ♊ .

Body ℂ , Cₒ .

Boil (v.) ✸ , ♏ .

Borax ⌂ , △ , ⌂ , ♃ , ♉ , ♉ , ♌ , ☽ , ℒₒ , ⱳ .

Brandy Ⅴ , ℬ , ♅ , „ , ⁰ₒ , ♯ .

Brandy, fruit   ⊕, 𝕏 .

Brandy, strongest possible   ℞ . 𝕍𝔸 .

Brass   ⚹, ♀, ♀, ♄, 5, ⊖, 𝕏, Ꙅ .

Brick dust   ⊡⊡⊡ , ⊡⊡ , ⊡⊡ ؛

Calcine (v.)   Ꞇ , Ꙅ , ẗ , ꭱ , Ꞓ , ⌣⌣ , ⌢⌢ , Z , エ .

Camphor   ∞∞∞∞ , ∞∞∞× , ∞∞× .

Cancer   ♋ .

Capricorn   ♑ .

Chalk   ♁ , ℓ .

Coagulate (v.)   ℓ , ℘ , ℊ , X X , Ʊ .

Coal   ↧ , ♁♁♁ .

Cobalt   ♂ .

Copper   ♀, ♀, ♀, ♀, ⊞, ⊡, ⚥, ⚹, ♃ , ⊼ .

Create a vacuum   2Ɔ .

Crucible   ♯ , ♯ , ♯ , ⚶ .

Crucible, melting   T , ₥ , ℓ , ℓ , ✗ .

Crystal   C , ℓ , Ꞓ , cƀ , cꜧ , H̃E , ⊕ , ℞ .

Day   ♂ .

Day and night   ♂♀, ♂♀ .

Death's Head (Caput Mortuum)   ☉ , ⊗ , ☉ , ☺ , ☽ , ✗ , ⌁ .

Decoction   ✗ .

Degree   ⌢ᵍ· .

Digest (v.) Δ. $\mathcal{D}\mathcal{G}$, $\mathcal{Z}\mathcal{Z}$, $\mathcal{Z}$, $\mathcal{Z}$.

Dissolve (v.) $\sim$, $\mathcal{S}^{\circ}$, $\mathcal{S}v$.,

Distill (v.) δ, $\mathcal{D}$, $\sim\mathcal{S}$, $\mathcal{D}$, $\maltese$, $\bar{o}$, $\mathcal{C}$, $\rightleftharpoons$, $\mathcal{D}m$., a, $\mathcal{C}\mathcal{D}$, $\mathcal{R}$

Distill in ash $\boxed{c}$.

Distill in sand $\boxed{:|:}$.

Dram 3, $3j$, $\mathcal{A}$.

Draw off $\mathcal{A}$.

Dry (adj.) $\int$.

Dry (v.) $\mathcal{D}$, D.

Drop (n.) $\mathcal{G}$. g, $g\mathcal{t}\mathcal{b}$.

Earth $\triangledown$, $\square$, $\mathcal{R}$, $\triangledown$.

Egg $\mathcal{L}$, $\bigcirc$.

Egg yolk χ, χ, $\overline{E}$.

Elements $\maltese$, E.

Emetic wine $\overline{E}$.

Equal amount of each $\overline{aa}$, $\bar{a}\bar{a}$, $\bar{a}$, $\widehat{aa}$, $\widehat{a \cdot a}$.

Essence $\maltese$, $\maltese$.

Ethyl alcohol V, K.

Ethyl alcohol, tartaric $\maltese$.

Extract (n.) H, X.

Fiat; become F, F.

Filter (v.) f, $\mathcal{P}$, 3, ∞, $\mathcal{O}w$, $\smile$.

Filter glass *f*3 .

Fire △, □, ⌡⌠, ⌡⌠, 𝘡o .

Fire, circulating △ᶜ, △, ⓒ, ▣ .

Fire, reverberating ℛ .

Fire, slow △⟩, ⌊△, △ .

Fire, strong △△, ⌢⌢ .

Fire grade ⌐⌐ .

Fix; coagulate (v.) ⇌, Ⅴ, ⋖, Ψ .

Flask ♂ .

Flour ⊙ .

Flow; melt (v.) F, ⸯ, ⸰, ⟿, o⸾ .

Fundamental matter ⌐⌐, ⸿, o ⅛ o .

Furnace ▢, ▣, ▣, ⊟, ⊖ .

Gemini ♊ .

Ginger ⟊⟊ .

Glass o⸮, o—o, ⊘, ⟆, ⨯, ⨯ .

Glass flask C, ♐, △ .

Glue ℒ, ∅, 𝒞 .

Glue, philosophical ℒ, ℱ, ℒ, ⌊ℕ, ℱ, ⸛ .

Gold ☉, ℞, ⸞, ⊙, △⟩, ⸴, ⋀, ⸞, ⟆ .

Grain *gr*, ℰ .

Gum; resin 𝒢, 9⸞9, ρ⸞ρ, ⌢⌢ .

Half ʃ./β .

Half a handful M/β .

Hartshorn C̲C̲ .

Hartshorn, burnt V̈ , V̊ , C C V .

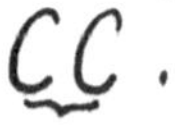

Herb Ħ , ƗB .

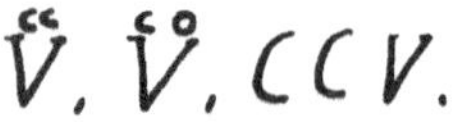

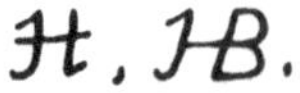

Herbal wine M .

Hermetically sealed Ħ , ƗB .

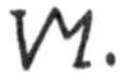

Hippocratic wine VH , V̵ .

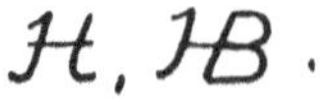

Honey M , M , ⚭ , ⬯ , ⚹ , ⚹ , ⊡ , ⊞ .

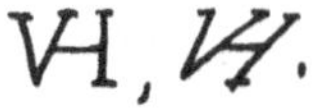

Horn C , ⨯ , ℓ .

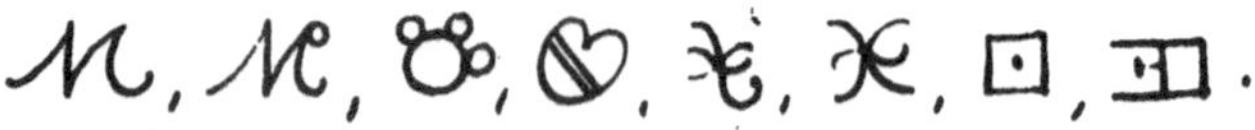

Horse dune C , ꝶ , C° , ₀°ꝍ , ꝑ° , Ψ , ⫫ , ⋏⋏ , ⸫ , Ꝗ

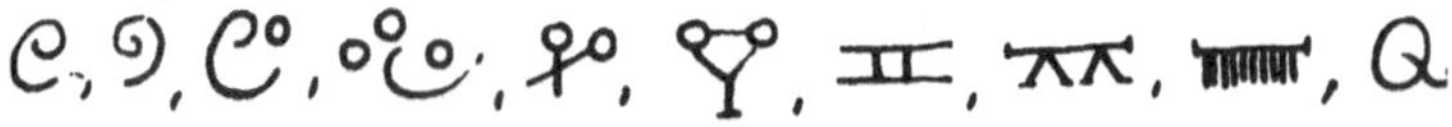

Hour ⚥ , Ə , ⊠ , ᚷ , ⊠ , ⊟ .

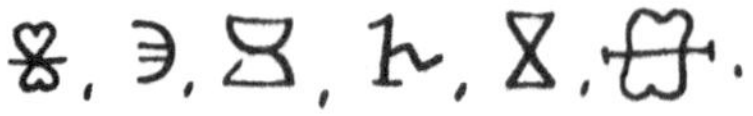

Imbibe ✡ .

Iron ♂ , o→ , ⋏ , ⇌ , ⤙ , ȝ , ⊡ .

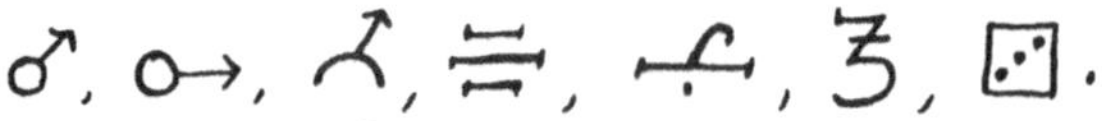

Juice; sap ⅋ , ⅋ .

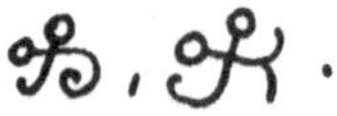

Lead (n.) ♄ , 5 , ¢ , c , ♄ , ⋏ , ℘ , P , ꝡ , ⋈ , ⧻ , ♄ .

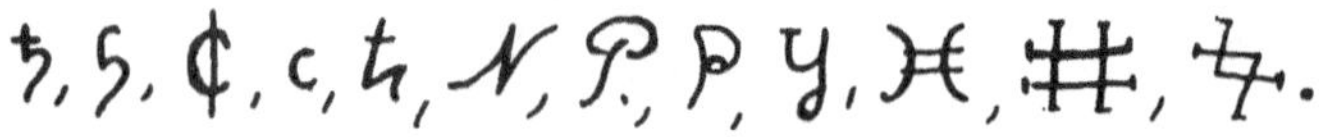

Leo ♌ .

Libra ♎ .

Liquefy (v.) ȝ , ≋ , m .

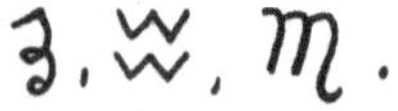

Lixiviate (v.) ⬳ .

Lye ⋇ , ♂ , ⴶ , � , ⟑ , 4⌣ , ℒ .

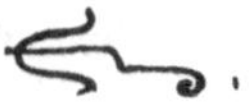

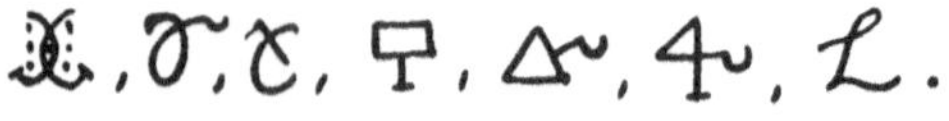

Lye of tartar ♀ .

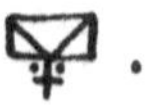

Magnesium o—ђ, ᘯ, Ð.

Matter ãã, maa.

Melt; fuse (v.) ⲧ, Ꞙ.

Mercury ☿.

Metal ♉, Ⴤ.

Mix (n.) ᘯ.

Mix together Ꝫↄ, Ꝭ.

Mixture ▲.

Month ʈʈ, ⤳, ⊠.

Moon, waning, decrescent ☾, ⏜.

Moon, waxing, crescent ☽, V̄.

Night ⌐, ∞.

Nutmeg ΛΥ.

Oil °°.

Oil, boiled °₀°.

Oil, common ₒₒ, ♂, ♌.

Oil, distilled ₒ°ₒ, ◉, ◍.

Oil, olive ℅, ₒ, ◉, ♇, ₒₒ.

Oil of tartar V, ♉, ♉, ◉, °₀°, 7, ¢.

Opposition ♂°.

Pebble; flint; silica °₀°.

Pisces ♓, ♓, ♓.

Potash; potassium carbonate Ψ, Ψ, Ψ, Ṫ, ⊡, ⊡, Ϭ, Ϥ, Χ, Χ.

Pound ⅄, ℔, ℔, ℃, ⚌, ℈, c. p.

Pound, apothecaries' m. p.

Pound, half ℔ 3, ℔⅓.

Powder (n.) Pulv., ℔.

Precipitate red ⚌ᵍᵗ·, r.

Precipitate, white ⚌, Ⴁ, ⚼ . .

Precipitated ⚌, ⚌ .

Prepare ℔, pp, p̃.

Pulverize Ꜫ, Ꜫ, ℗,)(, ⊶ .

Purification Ʋ, Ʋ, Ʋ, Ʋ, ₤.

Putrefaction ♈, ♈, ✝, ↔.

Quicklime ⚭, Ж, Χ, ℐ, ℭ, ℭ, ⚯.

Quicksilver (mercury) ☿, ☿, ☿, ₹, ℥, ⚌, ✝, ⚭, ℘, ⚭, ⟁, ♍, ⊡

Quintessence (Quinta Essentia) Q.E., ℉, Ɛ, qᵃ, qᵃ, 4ᵘ.

Quintessence of wine ⟂, ⟂, ℥, ╫.

Rain water ⚡, ▽, R▽, ▽, ▽.

Receptacle; receiver ℨ, ⟿.

Recipe ℞, Rec.

Reduction V, ⱳ, Ɛ.

Retort $\mathcal{C}$, $\mathcal{C}$, σ.

Reverberate R. $\mathcal{Z}$, ⚡.

Reverberating furnace ♄, ⊞ .

Root *Rad*.

Rub; pound; grind; triturate; grate ☿.

Saffron ⊕, $, $.

Sagittarius ♐.

Sal ammoniac ✳, ✳, ✳,)IC, ⦁⦁⦁⦁⦁, ╫╫╫, ☉,
⊥, ∞ .

Salt, common ⊖, $\mathcal{A}$, 7, ✗, □ .

Salt, rock 3, ⊡, ✧, ◻, 39, 61, 89 .

Salt, sea ⊕, ✗ .

Salt of tartar; fixed potassium carbonate ♀, ☺, ♀, ⊞ .

Salt of tartar saturated with vinegar ⊽, ⊻, ⊞,
□E, ℞.

Salt water ⊽.

Saltpeter ⊕, ⊙, ◐, ⊘, ♃, ⦁⦁⦁, ∞, ∧, ≋ .

Sand ⣿, ⣿, ⊟, S .

Scorpio ♏ .

Scruple), ♃, ℈ .

Scruple, half; obulus ℈β, ℮ .

Seal (n.) △ .

Seed; semen *ſem*.

Sextile ✳.

Simmer ⚸.

Smoke ⬿ , ⬿⬿ , ⬿⬿ , ♋ , ♉.

Soap ◇ , ♉.

Solve ♄ , ♄ , ♄ᵥ , E , Ė , Ē , ♈ , ♋ , 2 , ℥ , ℤ

Solvent ♀.

Solvent water ☥.

Soot; carbon black ✚ , △ , ℥.

Species *ſpec*.

Spirit ⌒ , ⌒ₛ , ⌒ₛ , ⚌ₛ , ⚌ , ⚌ , ⊶ ,

⊶ , ⊐⊏

Spring (season) ♃.

Steel ♂ , ♂ , ↔ , ♂⚹ , ♂ , ♄ , ♯.

Still (n.) ✗ , ✗.

Stones ✠ , ∈ , ♈.

Sublimate (n.) ♇ , ⚏ , 85 , S , ⋙.

Sublimate (v.) ⌐⌐ , ⌒ᵇ , ⚏ , ⋌.

Sugar Σ.

Summer ✳.

Tartar; hydrogen potassium tartrate ♀ , ⊞ , ♁ , ⊐ , ⫩

⊿⫪ , 63 , Ꮍ , ♂ , R , ℞.

Tartar emetic

Taurus

Test (n.)

Tin

Tincture

Tincture of tartar

Tinge

Tube; pipe

Until it is sufficient

Uric salts

Urine

Vinegar

Vinegar, distilled

Vinegar, thrice-distilled

Vinegar of red wine

Virgin soil

Virgin wax

Virgo; virgin

Volatile

Volatile salt

Warm

Water

Water, common $\vee$ mis , ⊞ .

Water, hot ▽ .

Water, spring ▽ont .

Water, tasteless ▽ , ⊩ .

Week ∑ .

Weeks, four ⊠ .

Weeks, three ▷⋈ .

Weeks, two ∑ ◁ .

Wind furnace ⊡ , ⊖ , ⊡ .

Wine ∨ , ☺ , ✗ , ✝ .

Wine, boiled ✔ .

Wine, circulated ⓥ , Ⓐ .

Wine, red ℝ , ℽ , ℣ .

Wine, sublimated ✔ .

Wine, white ⩕ , ∽ .

Winter ⫙ , ⌓ , ⌓ .

Without wine ∫ . v .

Wood ⚓ , ⚕ , ♄ .

Wool ⫛ .

Year ㉝ , ⧖ , ⟲ , ⊶ , ⊠ .

Yeast ⋇ , ⋈ .

Zinc ⅛ , ⒝ , ⊢⊣ , ⊞ .

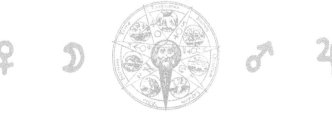

13
OLD WEIGHTS

The old pound varies between 327.5 and 360 grams. In Prussia, for instance, the pound had 350.78 grams. However, the relation between the pound valid in each case and the other weights usually remains constant. Here now follows a survey of the most important weights:

Grain	Scruple	Dram	Ounce	Pound	Gram
1	0.05	0.0167	0.0021	0.00017	0.0648
20	1	0.333	0.042	0.0035	1.296
60	3	1	0.125	0.0104	3.888
480	24	8	1	0.0833	31.103
5760	288	96	12	1	373.242

Further:

1 Obulus = 1/2 scruple = ℈β
  = 10 grains
1 Lot or Loth = 1/2 ounce = ℥β
  = 4 drams
𝓜, man., M, 𝓜 = 1 handful
β, 𝜷 behind a symbol means: half
  the amount, 𝓜j = 1 handful

𝓜β half a handful
ɿ, ı, j, ij = behind the symbol indicates the quantity
Mj = 1 handful
Mij = 2 handfuls
MijB = 2 1/2 handfuls
ãã = ana = an equal amount of each

247

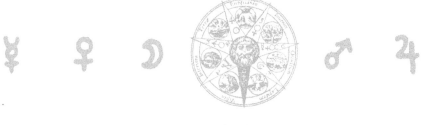

EPILOGUE
HOW CAN WE HEAL?

The condition of a sick person is always a condition of disorder, the proportions of the organism no longer being in balance.

The disturbed balance is either due to a deficiency or to an excess. Owing to the disturbed balance, the organism becomes prone to disease. By organism we here understand not only the physical constitution but also the etheric, astral, mental, and so forth.

A healthy organism in equilibrium ("a well-balanced organism") has greater resistance to infections; it knows how to defend itself in a natural way. An organism with a deficient balance finds it harder to resist attacks. It is like the control equilibrium in the Oriental martial arts.

What the sick organism lacks—for instance, minerals, vitamins, energies, trace elements, catalysts, and so on—must be supplied to it from outside, for example, from the plant, animal, or mineral world. What is present in dangerous excess must be broken down, driven out, or neutralized.

All the great classical schools of medicine consider right balance the foundation of health.

Chinese medicine stresses the necessary right proportion between the principles of Yin and Yang as well as between the Elements Fire, Earth, Metal, Water, and Wood as decisive for health. If the right proportion among these is disturbed, order is restored with both medicaments and acupuncture, or acupressure. This is the reason why acupuncture has also been called a therapy of order.[61]

In the view of Indian Āyurvedic medicine, the proportion between the *doṣas,* the *dhātus,* and the *malas* as well as the *mahābhūtas* is decisive for the state of health.

The three *doṣas,* Vāyu (Pneuma, air), Pitta (Chole, gall), and Kapha (Phlegma), whose true significance is to be understood in a much wider sense than their names, are above all responsible for the physico-chemical and physiological processes of the body, while the *dhātus* play the principal role in the formation of the body cells. The *malas* are substances that are partly absorbed within the body and partly eliminated in the form of feces, urine, and sweat after they have played their part.

Each of the *doṣas* contains the five *mahābhūtas* (protoelements). They are Ākāśa (space), Vāya (Air), Agni (Fire), Jala (Water), and Pṛthvi (Earth).

For obvious reasons, the Āyurvedic teaching already formulated a highly developed science of nutrition in the earliest times, which is still valid today. The teachings of Āyurveda were carried by Buddhist monks to other parts of the world. It strongly influenced Chinese as well as Greek and Arab medicine. Tibetan medical science is also founded on it.

The accuracy of the diagnosis of qualified Āyurvedic physicians is always amazing. During the International Congress on Traditional Asian Medicine at the Australian National University in Canberra,[62] to which I was summoned, the famous Tibetan physician of the Dalai Lama, L. Dölma, caused such a stir with the accuracy of her pulse diagnoses that some participants suspected a previous arrangement. It was only their own test that confirmed the extraordinary ability of this talented personage.

According to the views of ancient Greek medicine, too, the proportion between the fluids must be in balance. Hippocrates emphasizes this point in his humoral therapy.

An accurate diagnosis is a basic requirement for all these systems. The disease is always viewed in connection with the constitution of the patient. A famous Āyurvedic physician formulated it thus: we establish contact with each disease only through the patient.[63]

Patented broad-spectrum diagnoses are rarer in these therapeutic systems; mostly individually prescribed preparations are administered.

The defective balance of the organism becomes noticeable in various ways: a change in the body temperature, the condition of the different pulses that are felt at different spots, both on the surface and in depth, the condition and color of the skin, the eyes, the voice, the gait, the gesticulation, and the analysis of the urine and the blood are pointers. In occult medicine, the examination of the horoscope or the diagnostic pendulum—a doorway to the unconscious—is also used.

No doubt, modern Western medicine has made great progress, especially in surgery and technology. The ancients could not even dream of our modern cardiographs and encephalographs. Technology has led to important achievements in all areas; there are countless analyses at hand in our laboratories. But how is it that with all our scientific knowledge and analyses we can no longer build musical instruments like Stradivari and Guarneri? Everything in these instruments has been measured, analyzed, and examined—except that which cannot be analyzed. The result is sad, no end of single data, drawings, chemical analyses, and literature about violinmaking—but we cannot build a new Stradivarius, we are lacking something. "Thus he holds the parts in his hand, lacking, unfortunately, is the spiritual bond," Goethe instructed us. Caraka, one of the most important masters of Āyurvedic medicine, said: "A complete understanding of a science can never be attained if only a partial area of it is known." Essentially, both quotations are saying the same time. We know the message, but we do not act accordingly. What is it that makes the famous instruments of Cremona so unique? It is the sum of all proportions in perfect balance that bestows upon the instruments their exalted quality, not any tricks or details. The masters of Cremona, and also still much older masters who made outstanding lutes and base viols, worked with devotion and love, by "holy divine inspiration"; they were standing in "the light of Nature," to speak once more with Paracelsus. The same applies to great makers of Indian musical instruments. "*Dilse karna hay,"* one must build with the heart, a famous Indian instrument-maker once told the author.

If man does not try hard to recover his balance, a balance with himself, his fellow men, nature, and God, his life will become ever more misguided. This can already today be recognized by many symptoms of modern art, including the medical art.

The medicine of the future must find its way back to a great synoptic view; where the *Solve* only is achieved and not the *Coagula,* no true masters can emerge. Genuine alchemy belongs to the most precious and grand traditions, in comparison with which many concepts of modern science and technology appear spiritually impoverished.

There is really no reason for modern science to despise its venerable Mother Alchemy (Mater Alchymia).

It is only when man finds his way back to the whole that we can heal completely. As long as the parts behave as if they were the whole, the situation remains confused.

The same applies to politics and religions.

One of the noblest paths leading to a new synoptical view is alchemy, of which this modest work intends to give the reader an understanding.

Finally, let us remember an idea of Rudolf Steiner's: he said that the laboratory table must once again become an altar. With that everything is said. Have not the true alchemists acted in conformity with this all along? What would the world look like if the last-expressed thought were realized the world over? Perhaps we could then again make instruments of the caliber of Stradivari.

In conclusion, a bit of advice:

1. Before every experiment, you should mentally go through all the processes. Make sure that everything is at hand and that all your equipment is clean.
2. In distilling, take care of the necessary pressure compensation.
3. When distilling plant Sulfur, do not leave the tap at the oil separator open; it is a mistake that every alchemist makes at least once!

4. If you have to combine substances, first make a test with small amounts. If the reaction is violent, e.g., frothing over, join the substances slowly and carefully. In this way you will avoid quantitative losses.

5. Keep an orderly laboratory diary in which all dates, quantities, exact times, and the course of the experiment are exactly noted, including, of course, also all mistakes.

6. Avoid, especially at the beginning, all dangerous and poisonous substances.

7. Assess every preparation openly and critically. What matters is to become ever better in the spagyric art.

8. The laws on pharmacology and medicine in force in any specific country must be obeyed. Gather precise information about these so that you do not come into conflict with the law.

9. Let the keynote of your work be the desire to know the wonders of nature and the desire to help others. The highest form of medicine is love, says Paracelsus. If with his experiments the spagyrist does not at the same time devote himself to human spagyrics, that is, the perfecting of his personality, everything is but of little value.

10. Be aware that you are but an instrument of wise Nature and God.

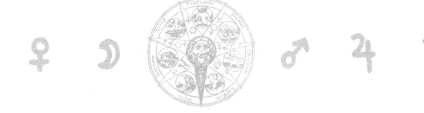

NOTES

1. A magistry (a masterpiece) is an alchemically exalted preparation that is always prepared from a whole, e.g., a medicinal plant. The preparation first requires the separation of specific constituents, after which they are purified and again combined.
2. See O. S. Johnson, *A Study in Chinese Alchemy* (Shanghai, 1928), and Ko Hung, *The Nei P'ien of Ko Hung: Alchemy, Medicine and Religion in the China of A.D. 320,* one of the ancient Chinese classical works of alchemy, translated by Prof. J. R. Ware.
3. Alchemy is especially strongly emphasized in South Indian medicine. The relevant texts have until now hardly been translated and are therefore practically only accessible in Tamil. According to information by Prof. R. Kumaraswamy (Govt. College of Indian Medicine, Palayamkottai), whom the author met at the International Congress on Asian Medicine at the Australian National University in Canberra in 1978, there are close parallels between Indian and Chinese medicine.
4. In the Western countries, Egyptian alchemy became the best-known tradition, so that alchemy was simply called the Hermetic art, after the god Thoth, better known as Hermes Trismegistus, the Thrice-Greatest Hermes.
5. Cf. E. J. Holmyard, *Alchemy,* p. 26, and M. Berthelot, *Collection des anciens alchimistes grecs.*
6. Until today, many modern representatives of Chinese medicine are holding on to ancient Chinese concepts, at least as a model, since no attempt at

explaining the phenomena of acupuncture on the basis of Western ideas has so far been entirely satisfactory.

7. Felix Mann, *Acupuncture: The Ancient Chinese Art of Healing and How It Works Scientifically* (New York, 1962).

8. *Ṛgveda* 1, 164.39.

9. Maharishi Mahesh Yogi.

10. Cf. Dr. Ch. H. Thakkur, *Āyurveda: Die indische Heil und Lebenskunst* (Freiberg, 1977), p. 224ff.

11. Bibliothèque de l'Arsenal, Paris, Ms. 974.

12. "Earth" here stands for everything that is impure and constitutes an unnecessary dead weight. (*Alchimia est separatio puri ab impuro:* Alchemy is the separation of the pure from the impure.) Here we must not confuse the word *earth* with the Element Earth, since the Elements can be purified. More about this later.

13. F. Hoyle, *Frontiers of Astronomy* (London, 1970), p. 304.

14. M. Capek, *The Philosophical Impact of Contemporary Physics* (Princeton, 1961), p. 319.

15. F. Capra, *The Tao of Physics* (London, 1978), p. 318.

16. In the meantime, this forecast has come true. Āyurvedic medicine is taught at several Indian universities. The Gujarat Āyurvedic University is devoting its entire curriculum exclusively to this subject. In addition, there are many Āyurvedic colleges and institutes proper.

17. *Spagyrische Arzneimittellehre* (Staufen Pharma, Göppingen, 1953), p. 112.

18. Paavo Airola, *How to Get Well* (Phoenix, Ariz., 1974), p. 140.

19. Louis Kervran, *Biological Transmutations* (Brooklyn, N.Y., 1972), p. 46.

20. The connection between alchemy and music is quite close. Many masters of alchemy were simultaneously musicians. Al-Razi, for instance, is also the author of an encyclopedia of music, at least it is ascribed to him. Indian classical music is directly a musical alchemy, aimed at the transformation of the listener's consciousness. ("A *rāga* is that which colors the mind" is a saying cited again and again.) The whole structure of a *rāga* in a concert proceeds according to the principle "Solve et Coagula." This range of the octave in which the *rāga* is anchored is divided into two parts, called *sthayi* and *antara*. These are separately developed in the introduction (*ālāpa*). The subsequent *sanchari* (wandering about) then joins the parts split by the Solve and that were separately elaborated. The *ālāpa* is largely analytical,

the single components are successively presented, only to be later once again incorporated into the whole. The composition (*bandish* or *gat*) following the introduction now brings the entire material into a firm form and can be compared to the alchemical fixation. In its structure the Solve is once more effected, leading thereafter to a blending that finally culminates in a vivacious, improvised embellishment developing from it.

21. Alexander von Bernus, *Alchymie und Heilkunst* (Nuremberg, 1972), pp. 95–96.
22. Nicolas Flamel, *Le Livre des figures hiéroglyphiques,* new ed. (Paris, 1971).
23. Raimundus Lullus, c. 1235–1315, Catalan alchemist and mystic.
24. Johannes Isaacus Hollandus, alchemist of the sixteenth–seventeenth century.
25. Tabula Smaragdina, in the alchemistic view, the legacy of Hermes Trismegistus, supposedly found in the Cheops pyramid. The text ranks as one of the fundamental hermetic confessions of faith, the Latin version of which runs as follows:

> Verum sine mendacio, certum et verissimum. Quod est inferius est sicut quod est superius, et quod est superius, est sicut est inferius, ad praeparanda miracula rei unius. Et sicut omnes res fuerunt ab uno, meditatione unius, sic omnes res natae fuerunt ab hac una re adoptione. Pater eius est Sol, Mater eius Luna. Portavit illud ventus in ventre suo. Nutrix eius terra est. Hic est vis totius mundi. Si versa fuerit in terram, separbis terram ab igne, subtile a spisso, suaviter cum magno ingenio. Ascendit a terra in coelum, et iterum descendit in terram, et recipit vim superiorum et inferiorum. Si habebis gloriam totius mundi. Ideo fugit a te omnis obscuritas, haed est totius fortitudinis fortitudo fortis, quae vincit omnem rem subtilem, et omne solidum penetrabit. Sic mundus creatus est. Hic erunt adoptiones mirabiles, quorum modus hic est, itaque vocatus sum Hermes Trismegistus, habens tres partes philosophiae totius mundi. Completum est quod dixi de operatione Solis.

> It is true without a lie, certain, and absolutely true. What is below is like what is above, and what is above is like what is below, so that the miracle of the One may be accomplished. And as all things have been from the One, so all things proceed from this One, by

adoption. Its father is the sun, its mother is the moon; the wind has carried it in his belly; its nurse is the earth.

This is the power of the whole world. If it is turned in the earth, you will separate the earth from the fire, the subtle from the dense, gently and with great cleverness. It ascends from the earth to heaven, and descends again to the earth and receives the power of Above and Below. So will you have the glory of the whole world.

Therefore, all darkness will flee from you. This is the mighty strength of all strength, which overcomes all things and transmutes every subtle thing and every coarse thing. Thus the world is created. From this will follow wonderful changes, the rules of which lie in this. Therefore I am called Hermes Trismegistus, having three parts of the philosophy of the whole world. It is ended now what I have said about the work of the sun.

26. *Hermetisches A.B.C. deren ächten Weisen alter und neuer Zeiten vom Stein der Weisen: Ausgegeben von einem wahren Gott und Menschenfreunde,* vols. 1 and 2 (Anstata, Schwarzenburg, 1979).

27. "Sammlung unterschieldich bewährter Chymischer Schriften, namentlich Joh." Isaaci Hollandi, Hand der Philosphen, Opus Saturni, Opera Vegeta-bilia, Opus Minerale, Cabala, de Lapide Philosophico, Nebst einem Tractat von den Irrgängen derer Alchymisten, Auctoris incerti, neue und verbes-serte Auflage, mit gehörigem Fleisse übersehen, und mit einem Verzeichnis derer in jeglichem Tractat befindlichen wichtigsten Materien vermehrt, wie auch mit nötigen Kupfern gezieret (Wien, Im Verlag bey Joh. Paul Krauss, Buchhändler, 1773).

28. Herrn Georgii von Welling, "Opus Mago-Cabbalisticum et Theosophicum, darinnen der Ursprung, Natur, Eigenschaften und Gerbrauch des Salzes, Schwefels und Mercurii, in dreyen Teilen beschrieben, und nebst sehr vielen sonderbaren mathematischen, theosophischen, magischen und mystischen Materien, auch die Erzeugung der Metallen und Mineralien, aus dem Grunde der Natur erwiesen wird; samt dem Haupt-Schlüssel des ganzen Werks, und vielen curieusen mago-cabbalistischen Figuren. Deme noch beygefüget: Ein Tractätlein von der Göttlichen Weisheit; und ein besonderer Anhang etlicher sehr rar- und kostbarer chymischer Piecen" (Frankfurt und Leipzig, in der Fleischerischen Buchhandlung, 1784; Reprint Stockholm, 1971).

29. Please do not play with *mantras*. According to tradition, they are extremely strongly acting vibrations. Their use should never be learned without the responsible instruction of a teacher.

30. Either longer or shorter verses of holy texts are designated as *mantras,* or the especially strongly effective monosyllabic *bijaksaras* (seed-syllables) or *bija-mantras* (seed-*mantras*). A *mantra* is a sound pattern (tone syllable form) whose effects are known. The *bija-mantras* all end in a nasal sound that is indicated by the point *(bindu),* also called *anusvara.* Right pronunciation sets the speaker vibrating and releases hidden powers. After correctly practicing with the spoken word, a mental repetition of the *mantra* is sufficient to bring about the effect. *Mantras* are an important aid to meditation.

31. Knorr von Rosenroth, *Aufgang der Arzney Kunst: Ortus Medicinae, of J. B. van Helmont* (reprint Munich, 1971), pp. 346, 352.

32. Helen Philbrick and Richard B. Gregg, *Companion Plants* (London, 1976), p. 73.

33. Alexander von Bernus, *Alchymie und Heilkunst* (Nuremberg, 1972), p. 122.

34. *Glauberus Concentratus* (Leipzig and Breslau, 1715), p. 7.

35. Cf. the instructions by D. J. Schroeder for the preparation of a spagyric essence from wormwood.

36. Cf. P. 72 of this work.

37. Archaeus: actually the *inwendige Werkmeister* (the inner master builder). An Archaeus can become volatile but not deteriorate. (See the work quoted in note 31, vol. 1, p. 40.) Great effects are ascribed to it. The water prepared as described represents the highest and stablest form of distilled water, which cannot be refined any further. As Archaeus in a narrower sense we designate an operating cause.

38/39. Theodor Kerckringii Doctoris Medici, *Anmerkungen über Basilii Valentini Triumphwagen des Antimonii* (Nuremberg, 1724), pp. 138, 206.

40. "Sammlung unterschiedlich bewährter Chymischer Schriften, namentlich Joh. Isaaci Hollandi Hand der Philosophen, Opus Saturni, Opera Vegetabilia, Opus Minerale, Cabala, de Lapide Philosophico, etc." (Vienna, 1773), p. 243.

41. According to Hollandus, the Sal Armoniacum ($*$ = ammoniac) unites substances even if they are opposed to each other by nature: "For without this Salt, no thing in the world will stay together nor come together." (See the

work cited in note 40, p. 212.) As the "Secret Salt of the Wise" it is one of the most important ingredients of certain preparations. Since ammoniac is extremely volatile, it is symbolically represented as an eagle. To collect the ammoniac, an "eagle trap" is used, a system of glass tubes in which the eagle gets stuck on its way during distillation, the Sal Armoniacum adhering to the walls of the tubes in the form of crystals.

42. Henry Monroe Fox, *Lunar Periodicity in the Reproduction of Centrichinus Setosus* (Royal Society of London, Series B), vol. XVCm, pp. 523–50.

43. L. Kolisko, *Sternenwirken in Erdenstoffen:* Saturn und Blei. Copyright 1952 by L. Kolisko, Edge near Stroud, England. Printed in Germany by J. M. Voith, GmbH, Heidenheim.

44. Michel Gauquelin, *Science and Astrology* (London, 1969).

45. John A. West and Jan G. Toonder, *The Case for Astrology* (Penguin Books, Harmondsworth, Middlesex, England).

46. The designation "Doctrine of Signatures" is understood in two ways: (1) Paracelsus says: "Nature marks every plant that issues from her for what it is good." Further: "And there is no thing in Nature created or born that does not also reveal its form externally; because the inner always works toward manifestation." Since balm has heart-shaped leaves, it is therefore considered marked as a cardiac remedy. (2) The assigning of certain plants to planets is also designated as Doctrine of Signatures, since the planets confer the Signum on plants.

47. Glauber, *Pharmacopoeia Spagyrica,* chap. 2.

48. Precise directions for the preparation of these distillates are found in the work *Ars Distillandi oder Destillierkunst dess wolerfahrnen Hieronymi Braunschweig.* This interesting work is published as a supplement to the edition of the herbal of Dioscurides of 1610 and also came out in 1964 as a reprint by Konrad Kölbl in Grünwald bei Munich.

49. Andreas Libavius, *Alchimiae Lib.* II, chap. 58.

50. According to Blakiston's *Medical Dictionary* (New York, 1979): Elixir: A sweetened, aromatic solution, usually hydroalcoholic, commonly containing soluble medicaments, but sometimes not containing any medication; intended for use only as a flavor or vehicle, or both.

51. L. Pomini in his work *Erboristeria Italiana,* on pectin: "In the human body they tone up the digestive tract and help neutralize poisonous wastes; in therapy they seem to be especially suited to correct excesses of gastric

acidity. They reduce the cholesterol content of the blood." (*Nei corpi umani tonificano l'intestino ed aiutano a neutralizzare i rifiuti venefici enterici; in terapia sembrano create apposta per correggere i difetti di acidità gastrica. Abbassano il tasso di colesterolo nel sangue.*)

52. Andreas Libavius, Lib. 2, *Alchimiae Tract. 3, De Specibus Compositis.*
53. Johannes Baptista Porta, *Magiae naturalis libri viginti* (Leiden, 1651), p. 439.
54. History and description of influential, elemental, and natural effects / Of all foreign and native plants / also of their subtlety / together with their true and artificial counterfeiting / also of all parts / internal and external members of the human body / in addition to an illustration of all instruments for their extraction / likewise their use / and all processes necessary for the preservation of health. Described by Leonhardt Thurneysser zum Thurn, Appointed Electoral Brandenburg Medicus in ordinary. Reprinted by Arcana S. Schmidt Verlag, Handeloh, 1978.
55. Le Febure, *Neuvermehrter chymischer Handleiter und guldenes Kleinod* (Nuremberg, 1685), p. 343.
56. Andreas Libavius, Lib. 2, *Alchimiae Tract. 3, De Specibus Compositis.*
57. Alkali is the Salt extracted through the calcination of a whole plant. To this end, the closed calcination is suggested, which Libavius also advises.

 In the preparation of the alkalis, the salts are extracted as much as possible with the plant's "own water," i.e., with the water of the plant carefully distilled through heating and then made visible through slow evaporation. Otherwise, spring water is recommended for the extraction of the salts. Libavius describes the process in his Lib. 2, *Alchimiae Tract. 2, De Extractis:* The alkali, however, arises out of the total essence of the substances, so that it carries with itself the inner powers, while only the Corpus is separated. It is extracted from vegetable, animal, and mineral substances that are all together reverberated in ash or lime, during which the container must be closed as much as possible and the joints sealed to prevent even a trace of essence from escaping, and to keep the volatile together with the fixed.
58. Johannes Baptista Porta, *Magiae naturalis libri viginti,* p. 439.
59. *Johannes Isaaci Hollandi Opus Vegetabile,* by his son Sendivogius, known as J.F.H.S., published by Henrico Betkio, Amsterdam, 1659.
60. In chapter 30 of his *Opus Vini,* Hollandus describes the combustible or bad-smelling oil as hot and moist: "This combustible oil which you have

just rectified is now clear, thin, and red, like blood, also fat like other oil, and it is hot and moist. It is good for chilled and gouty nerves, to rub or anoint them with, also for paralyzed and frozen members, likewise for those who have an apoplectic stroke. It also serves in all ointments and poultices to 'incarnate' or make the flesh grow in all deep holes and wounds." In chapter 31, he warns the physicians of any misuse of the oil: "If a master or surgeon intending to heal a wound puts too much fat oil in to the ointment, the flesh will imperceptibly become too rank, and bad flesh will grow in it, and if he continues with the same ointment, not making it leaner, it will result in corruption and putrefaction in the nerves and the flesh, so that finally fistulas, cancer, and running holes will arise in it. All this is caused by the combustible oil which they have extracted from the earth, and thus it becomes clear that the combustible oil can also cause death."

61. Gerhard Bachmann, *Die Akupunktur—eine Ordnungstherapie* (Karl F. Haug Verlag, Heidelberg, 1959).

62. International Conference on Traditional Asian Medicine (ICTAM), Australian National University, Canberra, 2–7 September 1979, under the auspices of the World Health Organization. This congress, suggested by Prof. L. Basham, the first of its kind, turned into an epoch-making success. It resulted in the foundation of IASTAM (International Association for the Study of Traditional Asian Medicine, Inc.) with Prof. Basham as president. The goal of IASTAM is to realize and further develop the suggestions resulting from the Congress. Other congresses are planned for the future. In the meantime, the organization counts many prominent members throughout the world.

63. The famous Āyurvedic physician Pundit Shiv Sharma, in the course of a conversation with the author.

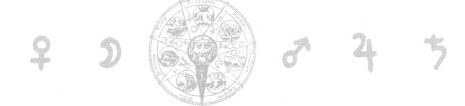

BIBLIOGRAPHY

Agrippa von Nettesheim. *Magische Werke,* 2 vols. Reprint Ansata-Verlag, Schwarzenburg, 1979.

Albertus, Frater. *The Alchemist of the Rocky Mountains.* Paracelsus Research Society, Service Press, Inc., Salt Lake City, Utah, 1976.

———. *The Alchemists Handbook.* Samuel Weiser, New York, rev. ed., 1974.

———. *Praktische Alchemie im zwanzigsten Jahrhundert.* Paracelsus Research Society, Salt Lake City, Utah, 1970.

Astrologia oggi, a cura di Serena Foglia. Armenia Editore, Milan, 1976.

Barbault, André. *Traité pratique d'astrologie.* Editions du seuil, Paris, 1961.

Barbault, Armand. *L'oro del millesimo mattino.* Italian translation by Stefania Binarelli, Biblioteca dei misteri, diretta da Gianfranco de Turris. Edizioni Mediterranée, Rome, 1972. (Publications Premieres, Paris, 1969.)

Bernus, Alexander von. *Alchemie und Heilkunst.* Verlag Hans Carl, Nuremberg, 1969 and 1972.

Bersetz, J., and A. Masson. *Traité de spagyrie.* Editeur J. B. G., Paris, VIII, 1977.

Besesti, Violetta. *Astrologia lunisolare,* Casa Editrice MEB, Turri, 1975.

Bhagavad Gitā. Triest, 1975.

Cecchini, Tina. *Enciclopedia delle erbe e delle piante medicinali.* De Vecchi Editore, Milan. 1977.

Cornell, H. L., M.D. *Encyclopedia of Medical Astrology.* 3rd rev. ed. Samuel Weiser, New York, 1972.

Da Legnano, Dott., P. L. *Le piante medicinali nella cura delle malattie umane,* 3rd ed., rev. Edizioni Mediterranée, Rome, 1973.

Dash, Dr. Bhagwan. *Fundamentals of Āyurvedic Medicine.* Bansal & Co., New Delhi, 1978.

———. *Āyurveda for Healthy Living.* Hind Pocket Books, New Delhi, 1977.

Dash, Dr. Bhagwan, and Manfred M. Junius. *A Handbook of Āyurveda.* Concept of Publishing Co., New Delhi, 1983.

Deichmann, Hilmar M. D. *Catena Medica.* Karl F. Haug Verlag, Heidelberg, 1976.

Dioscurides. *Kreutterbuch.* Frankfurt, 1610. Reprint Konrad Kölbl, Grünwald near Munich, 1964.

Evola, Julius. *La tradizione ermetica.* 5th ed. Edizioni Mediterranée, Rome, 1971.

Fankhauser, Dr. Alfred. *Das wahre Gesicht der Astrologie.* 3rd ed. Orell Füssli Verlag, Zurich, 1952.

———. *Horoskopie.* 2nd ed. Orell Füssli Verlag, Zurich, 1946.

Fischer, Georg. *Heilkräuter und Arzneipflanzen.* Karl F. Haug Verlag, Berlin-Tübingen-Saulgau, 1947; 4th ed., 1975.

Fyfe, Agnes. *Die Signatur des Mondes im Pflanzenreich.* Kapillardynamische Untersuchungsergebnisse. Verein für Krebsforschung, Arlesheim, Switzerland. Verlag Freies Geistesleben, Stuttgart, 1967.

Gessman, G. W. *Die Geheimsymbole der Chemie und Medizin des Mittelalters.* Graz, Publ. by the author, 1899. Exact reprint of the 1899 edition. Dr. Martin Sändig, oHG. Walluf bei Wiesbaden, 1972.

Glauberus Concentratus. Leipzig and Breslau, 1715. Publ. Michael Hubert, reprint 1961, Karl F. Haug Verlag, Ulm/Donau.

Hahnemann, Samuel. *Organon der Heilkunst,* "Aude Sapere," 6th ed. Karl F. Haug Verlag, Heidelberg, 1981.

Heindel, Max, and Augusta Foss-Heindel. *Astro-Diagnose: Ein Führer zur Heilung.* Rosenkreuzer Gemeinschaft, Darmstadt, 1969.

Helmrich, Dr. Hermann E. *Spagyrik: Alter Wein in neuen Schläuchen.* Karl F. Haug Verlag, Heidelberg, 1977.

Hermetisches A.B.C., 2 vols. Reprint Ansata Verlag, Schwarzenburg, 1979, in accordance with the Berlin edition of 1778.

Hollandus, Johannes Isaac. *Opera Vegetabilia.* In Sammlung unterschiedlich bewährter Chymischer Schriften, Publ. by Joh. Paul Krauss, Vienna, 1773.

Holmyard, E. J. *Storia dell-alchimia.* Sansoni, Florence, 1959.

Karl, Josef. *Phytotherapie.* Publ. Tibor Marczell, Munich, 1978.

Kervran, C. Louis. *Biological Transmutations.* Crosby Lockwood, London, 1972.

———. *A la découverte des transmutations biologiques, une explication des phénomènes biologiques aberrants.* Le Courier du Livre, Paris, 1966.

———. *Preuves relatives à l'existence de transmutations biologiques, échecs en biologie a la loi de Lavoisier d'invariance de la matière.* Maloine, Paris, 1968.

———. *Les transmutations biologiques en agronomie.* Maloine, Paris, 1970.

———. *Alchimie d'hier et d'aujourd'hui: L'alchimie, rêve ou réalité.* Revue des Ingénieurs de l'Institut National Supérieur de Rouen, 1972–73.

Kinauer Saltarini, Helen. *Gli astri e la salute.* Giovanni De Vecchi Editore, Milan, 1976.

Kolisko, L. *Sternenwirken in Erdenstoffen:* Saturn und Blei. Ein Versuch, die Phänomene der Chemie, Astronomic und Physiologic zusammen zu schauen. Copyright 1952 by L. Kolisko. Edge near Stroud, England. Printed in Germany by J. M. Voith GmbH, Heidenheim.

Kurth, Hanns. *Rezepte berühmter Ärzte aus 5000 Jahren.* Ramón F. Keller Verlag, Geneva, 1974.

Le Febure. *Neuvermehrter chymischser Handleiter und guldenes Kleinod.* Nuremberg, 1685.

Libavius, Andreas. *Alchemia.* Andreae Libavii Med. D. Poet. Physici Rotemburg, Exudebat Johannes Saurius, Impensis Petri Kopfii, Frankfurt, 1597.

———. *Alchemia: Commentari I* (2nd ed. of *Alchemia*). Exudebat Johannes Saurius, Impensis Petri Kopfii, Frankfurt, 1606.

Die Alchemie des Andreas Libavius. Ein Lehrbuch der Chemie aus dem Jahre 1597. Verlag Chemie, Weinheim, 1964.

Mességué, Maurice. *Die Natur hat immer recht.* Molden, Vienna, 1973.

———. *Die Kräuter meines Vaters.* Molden, Vienna, 1974.

———. *Von Menschen und Pflanzen.* Molden, Vienna, 1972.

Ming Wong. *La médecine chinoise par les plantes.* Edition Tschou, 1976.

Monroe Fox, Henry. *Lunar Periodicity in the Reproduction of Centrichinus Setosus.* Royal Society of London, Series B, vol. XVCm, p. 523–50.

Musaeum Hermeticum Reformatum et Amplificatum. Akademische Druck und Verlagsanstalt, Graz, 1970.

Negri, G. *Nuovo erbario figurato.* Ulrico Hoepli Editore, Milan, 1976.

Paoli, Alberto. *Introduzione all'astrologia.* Giovanni De Vecchi Editore, Milan, 1973.

Paracelsus. *The Hermetic and Alchemical Writings of Paracelsus,* edited by Arthur Edward Waite. Reprint of the 1894 edition published by James Elliot & Co., London. Shambhala Publications, Berkeley, Calif., 1976.

———. *Sämtliche Werke,* nach der zehnbändigen Huserschen Gesamtausgabe (1589–1591) zum ersten Mal in neuzeitliches Deutsch übersetzt. Mit Einleitung, Biographie und erklärenden Anmerkungen versehen von Bernhard Aschner. 4 vols. Jena, 1926–1932.

Pelikan, Wilhelm. *Heilpflanzenkunde,* vols. 1, 2, and 3. Philosophisch-Anthroposophischer Verlag, Dornach, 1975.

Quinta Essentia, journal of alchemy, astrology, Kabbalah. Paracelsus Research Society, P.O.B. 8, CH-6414, Oberarth, Switzerland.

Ranque, Georges. *La pietra filosofale.* Italian translation by Vincenzo Montenegro, Biblioteca dei misteri, diretta da Gianfranco de Turris. Edizione Mediterranée, Rome, 1973. (Editions Robert Laffont, Paris, 1972).

Ring, Thomas. *Astrologie ohne Aberglauben.* Econ Verlag, Düsseldorf-Vienna, 1972.

———. *Astrologische Menschenkunde,* vols. 1–4. Rascher Verlag, Zurich and Stuttgart, from 1956.

Knorr von Rosenroth, Christian. *Aufgang der Artzney-Kunst,* 2 vols. Kösel Verlag, Munich, 1971.

Sadoul, Jacques. *Il tesoro degli alchimisti.* Italian translation by Jacopo Comin, Bibliotheca dei misteri, diretta da Gianfranco de Turris. Edizioni Mediterranée, Rome, 1972. (Editions Publications Premiers ed Editions "J'ai lu," Paris, 1970.)

Schatzkammer der Alchemie. Fontes Artis Chymicae. Akademische Druck und Verlagsanstalt, Graz, 1976.

D. Johann Schröders trefflich / versehene Medizin / Chymische Apotheke / Oder: Höchstkostbarer Arzeney-Schatz, 2 vols. Nuremberg, 1685. Reprint 1963, Konrad Kölbl, Grünwald bei Munich.

Scoprire niconoscere usare le erbe. Fratelli Fabbri Editore, Milan, 1977. Consulente: Paolo Rovesti, testi di Umberto Boni e Gianfranco Patri, tavole di Alessandro Bartolomelli.

Sementowsky-Kurilo, Nikolaus von. *Astrologie, Schicksal im Sternenspiegel.* Aurum Verlag, Frieburg i. Br., 1979.

Spagyrische Arzneimittel-Lehre. Staufen Pharma, Göppingen, 1938, 1953.

Tabernaemontanus, Jacobus Theodorus. *Neu vollkommen Kräuterbuch*. Frankfurt, 1610. Reprint Konrad Kölbl, Grünwald bei Munich, 1964.

Thakkur, Vaidyaratna Chandrasekhar, G. *Introduction to Āyurveda*. ASI Publications, Inc., New York, 1974. German translation by Dr. Ulrike Killer.

Vaga, Eugenio, G. *Dottor Natura: Malattia per malattia, le ricette erboristiche che curano e guariscono*. De Vecchi Editore, Milan, 1974.

Valentinus, Basilius. *Chymische Schriften*. 2 vols. Hamburg, 1677 bei Johann Naumanns and Dr. H. A. Gerstenberg, Hildesheim, 1976.

———. *Triumphwagen des Antimons*, mit dem Kommentar des Theodor Kerckringius. Amsterdam, 1685.

Valnet, Jean. *Aromatherapie: Traitement des maladies par les essences des plantes*. 8. Maloine Editeur, 1976.

Vitofranceschi, Giuseppe de. *L'aglio, una pianta medicinale da riscoprire*. Paracelso, Collana di Fitoterapia a cura del Prof. Giuseppe de Vitofranceschi, Mario Solfanelli Editore, Chieti, 1978.

Welling, G. v. *Opus Mago-Cabbalisticum et Theosophicum*. Leipzig, 1784. Reprint C. Wendelholm, Stockholm, 1971.

West, John Anthony, and Jan Gerhard Toonder. *The Case for Astrology*. Macdonald, 1970. Penguin Books, Harmondsworth, Middlesex, England.

Willfort, Richard. *Gesundheit durch Heilkräuter*. Rudolf Trauner Verlag, Linz, 1977.

Zolla, Elémire. *Le Meraviglie della natura*. Introduzione all'alchimia, Bompiani, Milan, 1975.

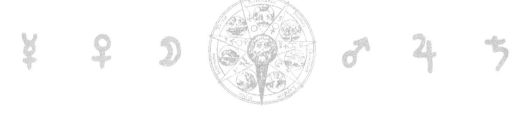

SPAGYRIC RESOURCES

Publisher's note: These resources were added to the 2007 edition to alert readers to some of the products and information available about spagyrics. While certainly not all-inclusive, these sites represent the range of spagyric material available online.

The Alchemy Web Site
Glasgow, United Kingdom
http://www.levity.com/alchemy/home.html

Run by Adam McLean, provides links to alchemical texts, images, bibliographies, study courses, and a bookstore. Hosts the discussion group Alchemy Academy, for those interested in more scholarly research.

Alchemystica
http://tech.groups.yahoo.com/group/alchemystica/

Provides a platform for discussion of subjects ranging from laboratory techniques to inner spiritual practice, drawing from both Eastern and Western traditional works on alchemy.

Al-Kemi

Walterville, Oregon

http://www.al-kemi.com

Offers spagyric essences, magisteries, initiatics, somalixir-spiritualized formulas, erosoma nectars of love, and custom elixirs. Also provides background information explaining the physical, energetic, and initiatic characteristics of alchemy.

Australerba Herbal Products & Spagyric Laboratories

Ridleyton, Australia

http://australerba.com.au/home.html

Manfred Junius was a founding partner of this company. This site includes product descriptions, production details, and testimonials.

Crucible Catalog

Sacramento, California

http://www.crucible.org

Offers alchemical products including artwork, esoteric equipment, hermetic arts, tinctures and elixirs, meditation supplies, and laboratory equipment.

Spagyrium: Alchemical Elixirs, Tinctures & Tonics

http://www.spagyrium.com

An online store where you can purchase spagyric elixirs, tinctures, tonics, and salts. Also provides a list of alchemy resources.

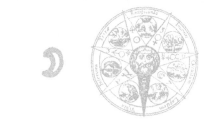

INDEX

undulation, Mercury corresponding to, 33
until it is sufficient, symbol for, 245
uranium, 17
Urbigerus, Baron, *Circulatum Minus,* 163–80
uric salts, symbol for, 245
urine, symbol for, 245
"Usefulness" (Valentinus), 26

Valentinus, Basilius, 23–28
   Triumphal Chariot of Antimony, 84, 23
   Twelve Keys of Hermetic Philosophy, 23, 22
valerian, 130–31
van der Doost, Paulus, 27, 28
Vāya, 250
Vāyu, 250
Vegetable Stone. *See* Plant Stone
Venus, plants under the Dominion of, 107–10
vinegar
   distillation of, 84
   symbol for, 245
violinmakers, 4
virgin soil, symbol for, 245
virgin wax, symbol for, 245
Virgo, 245, 126
Viridarium Chymicum, 23, 31–33
volatile, symbol for, 245
volatilizing alkaline Salts, 176
von Bernus, Alexander, 20
   Alchymie und Heilkunst, 33, 20
   Hieroglouphicic Figures, 33
von Hohenbeim, Theophrastus Bombastus. *See* Paracelsus

von Welling, Georg, *Opus Mago-Cabbalisticum et Theosophicum,* 45–46
Vries, Hans Fredemann, 27, 28
Vulcan, 27

warm, symbol for, 245
water, 37–38
   symbol for, 245–46
water-bath, 77
water buffalo's milk, 10
week, symbol for, 246
weights, 247–49
West, Horn Anthony, 97
Western medicine, 251
Western pharmacology, 7–8
"Wet Way," 168
wheat, 10
wind furnace, symbol for, 246
windmill (Victoria), 21
wine, 168, 219–33
   symbol for, 246
winged snake, 27
winter, symbol for, 246
wood, symbol for, 246
Word of God, 42

yang, 42
year, symbol for, 246
yeasts, 54
   symbol for, 246
yin, 42

Zimpel, Carl Friedrich, 19–20
zinc, symbol for, 246
zodiac, 127, 126–29
   See also astrology; planets
Zosimos of Panopolis, 2